Respiratory and Alimentary Tract Diseases

Perspectives in Pediatric Pathology

Vol. 11

Series Editors
Harvey S. Rosenberg
Professor of Pathology and Pediatrics,
University of Texas Medical School, Houston, Tex.
Jay Bernstein
Director of Anatomic Pathology,
William Beaumont Hospital, Royal Oak, Mich.

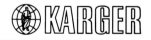

Basel · München · Paris · London · New York · New Delhi · Singapore · Tokyo · Sydney

Respiratory and Alimentary Tract Diseases

Volume Editors
Harvey S. Rosenberg, Houston, Tex.
Jay Bernstein, Royal Oak, Mich.

110 figures and 15 tables, 1987

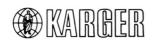 KARGER

Basel · München · Paris · London · New York · New Delhi · Singapore · Tokyo · Sydney

Perspectives in Pediatric Pathology

Library of Congress Card No. 72–88828

© Copyright 1987 by S. Karger AG, P.O. Box, CH–4009 Basel (Switzerland)
Printed in Switzerland by Boehm-Hutter AG, Reinach BL
ISBN 3–8055–4435–9

Contents

Preface

With a focus on the respiratory and digestive systems, this volume also presents a biography of Agnes Rose Macgregor (1894–1982), whose early contributions to the pathology of bacterial pneumonia set standards that still apply. Her life spanned the emergence of pediatric pathology from a low-yield, idle curiosity, through a phase of discovery and inventory, to its current status as a discipline worthy of lifelong study. Her initial, almost casual, introduction to pediatric pathology led to the establishment of the renowned Department of Pathology at the Royal Hospital for Sick Children in Edinburgh and the training of some of the current leaders in the field. Her discussion of pulmonary hyaline membranes [Macgregor, A.R.: *Pathology of Infancy and Childhood*, Livingstone, Edinburgh 1960] expressed her skepticism of the 30-year-old concept that the membranes originated from aspirated vernix caseosa, and she supported the then recent recognition of their endogenous origin. In his chapter on the pathology of neonatal surfactant deficiency, Robertson provides key links in understanding the pathogenesis of neonatal respiratory distress by his focus on alveolar physics, experimental models, and the therapeutic approach of surfactant replacement.

The several disorders and processes resulting in diffuse pulmonary hemorrhage and hemosiderosis provide a challenge to diagnosis and prognosis. In his chapter on idiopathic pulmonary hemosiderosis in the first decade of life, Cutz outlines the features that distinguish the idiopathic condition from pulmonary hemosiderosis secondary to other, usually systemic diseases. Landing (in the first of 2 manuscripts in this volume) illustrates the special features of pulmonary hemosiderosis associated with thalassemia major in which iron deposition in the pulmonary connective tissue appears to explain the reduced pulmonary compliance in some patients.

During the last decade, esophageal biopsy has emerged as a common procedure in several esophageal inflammatory disorders, particularly in esophagitis due to gastroesophageal reflux and in Barrett's esophagus. The chapters by Dahms and Rothstein and by Groben and her colleagues identify the clinical, physiologic, and histologic criteria for relating esophageal inflammation to gastroesophageal reflux and the potential for medical or surgical management.

Landing once again provides a new way of looking at things. In flat, whole-mount preparations, Landing and his colleagues demonstrate and provide a basis for quantitating the Auerbach plexus of the human gastrointestinal tract. They illustrate the peculiar anatomy of the intestinal nervous plexus which allows for preservation of the geometry while accomodating to changes in dimension of the gut during dilatation and contraction.

This volume finishes with two childhood disorders that have a geographic distribution. Joshi describes Indian Childhood Cirrhosis with its apparent selective localization to India. Its pathogenesis is not understood, although it may be related to exogenous copper from the use of copper-based containers and cooking utensils. The intestinal pseudo-obstruction due to degenerative leiomyopathy described by Kaschula and his colleagues in indigenous Africans only superficially resembles the similarly named disorder encountered in western countries. Although pseudo-obstruction and muscle degeneration of the gastrointestinal tract dominate the syndrome, the degeneration apparently affects blood vessels, the urinary tract and the lung.

Once again, the editors are thankful for the hard working Board of Editors, our unsung ad hoc reviewers, our publishers, and most of all the intellectual stamina and resilience of the individual authors for persisting against time and adversity in getting out their messages.

H.S.R.
J.B.

Board of Editors

Perspect. pediatr. Pathol., vol. 11, pp. 1–5 (Karger, Basel 1987)

Founders of Pediatric Pathology:
Agnes Rose Macgregor, MD, FRCPE, FRCOG

Former Reader in the Pathology of the Diseases of Infancy and
Childhood in the University of Edinburgh, and Consultant
Pathologist to the Royal Hospital for Sick Children, Edinburgh and
the South-East Scotland Regional Hospital Board[1]

Douglas Bain

Department of Genetic Pathology, Royal Hospital for Sick Children and Honorary
Senior Lecturer, Department of Pathology, University of Edinburgh, UK

Agnes Macgregor's first experience of Pathology in a children's hospital was in 1918 when, having completed the Pathology course and her
third undergraduate year in Edinburgh University, she was asked by Professor J. Lorrain Smith to perform post-mortem examinations and report
biopsies and bacteriological specimens for a few months at the Royal Hospital for Sick Children, whose pathologist was then away on war service.
This she did, on a part-time basis, for 6 months during a summer term and
vacation. The hospital's rudimentary pathology service gave Agnes a first
insight into paediatric pathology.

In 1920 she graduated MB, ChB at Edinburgh University. In 1922,
when she had joined the staff of the University Pathology Department
under Professor Smith, she returned to the Children's Hospital as part-

---

[1] Editors Note: In preparing for this biography, Dr. Bain had asked Dr. Macgregor for
a few notes about her career. Dr. Macgregor's notes, written in the third person, reached
Dr. Bain just about a week before she died and appear here as her biography. The last four
paragraphs of the text formed the basis of her obituary in the *Lancet* of Saturday, February
27, 1982, reproduced here with the permission of the Editors [1].

Of Dr. Macgregor's photograph, Dr. Bain writes: 'I enclose a photograph of Agnes
taken in the early 1950s with Kitty Dye, the family cat of the first proven case of congenital
toxoplasmosis in the UK [2]. We brought Kitty Dye over for investigation, but unfortunately
our technology in those days was not enough to confirm our suspicions that the cat was a
source of infection.'

time pathologist and bacteriologist, and thereafter retained her close association with paediatric pathology until her retirement in 1960.

In 1924 the Elsie Inglis Memorial Maternity Hospital was opened, replacing the old Hospice in High Street. At that time the medical staff there were all women, as one of the objectives of the hospital was to provide facilities for women doctors, who were excluded from other hospitals. With no other woman pathologist in the Edinburgh area, Agnes was asked to provide laboratory services. Although numbers were small, the work provided Agnes with her first experience in perinatal pathology.

Increased experience came in the 1930s, when she was appointed part-time pathologist to the Simpson Memorial Maternity Pavilion, which was built in the grounds of the Royal Infirmary to replace the old hospital in Lauriston Place. Agnes received little help from colleagues, partly because no one knew much about perinatal pathology and partly because of skepticism about its usefulness. Post-mortems after perinatal deaths were considered useless because nothing could be found, and bacteriological examinations were useless because of post-mortem contamination. After a long struggle, Agnes refuted the first as untrue and the second as avoidable by careful technique. She had been particularly impressed with the importance of infection in perinatal mortality, and in 1939 her report [3] on pneumonia in the newborn did much to convince the skeptics. She showed, against much opposition, that the gram-negative coliform bacilli were among the most frequent pathogens in perinatal infections, especially in gastroenteritis and meningitis.

Although perinatal pathology became Agnes's chief occupation, it was never the only one; she retained close contact with diseases of older children. Until her retirement, Agnes maintained an interest in tuberculosis [4–6] which had been aroused as an undergraduate by Sir Robert Phillip, and continued for many years. As hospitals with children's and maternity wards became interested, she received requests for help, culminating in the supervision of a paediatric pathology service throughout the South-East Region of Scotland, mainly after the introduction of the National Health Service, and with the invaluable help of her successive assistants, Kenneth Rhaney, Albert Claireaux and Douglas Bain.

During the whole of Agnes's tenure of these positions, her work was hampered by two serious shortages, space and money. When she began her short undergraduate adventure in 1918 the Pathology Department at the Royal Hospital for Sick Children consisted of one small room in the Radiology Department behind the hospital, which housed a part-time

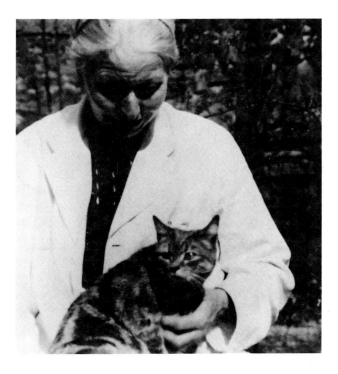

pathologist, a part-time technician, a postmortem room and a preparation room. When, in the 1920s, the Radiology Department required the room, new premises were provided by building a second floor above the old block, providing two small rooms, one for the pathologist and one for the technician. When the demands on the Department increased further, the same two rooms housed an assistant pathologist, an assistant technician, and later, a secretary. This was in the time of the voluntary hospitals when Boards of Directors had difficulty finding money for extension of buildings or new equipment. With the introduction of the National Health Service, this problem was solved to some extent, but the cumbersome administration sometimes caused frustrating delays, and much depended on the goodwill of local hospital committees.

Dr. Agnes Macgregor died on Wednesday, 20th January, 1982, in Glen Lyon, aged 88. As a daughter of the Manse[2], her personality was

[2] A daughter of the Manse is a minister's daughter. Dr. Macgregor's father was a minister in the Church of Scotland.

such that she was respected and admired by all those who had the privilege of working with her. She was one of the pioneers of pathology in a world which still refused to accept the role of women in medicine. Her struggle was unique. Dr. Agnes was one of the first doctors to draw attention to the importance of pathology in determining the causes of infant and childhood mortality. She worked in close association with the late Sir Robert Phillip and afterwards with Sir John Crofton, both pioneers in the fight against tuberculosis. She had wholehearted support from such eminent pathologists as Prof. J. Lorrain Smith and Prof. J.M. Drennan and also from Prof. Charles McNeil, the first Professor of Child Life and Health in Scotland. As an internationally recognized expert in her subject she established in Edinburgh a school of paediatric pathology and the unique Department of Paediatric Pathology at the Royal Hospital for Sick Children in Edinburgh which has world wide recognition.

Not only was Dr. Macgregor a pioneer in baby pathology but she was the first lady Elder of the Church of Scotland. She presented the chalice to the Queen at the Communion in St. Giles in 1968. To commemorate that event the congregation of Glen Lyon presented to the Queen Communion tokens dating back to the 18th Century and which the Queen was delighted to accept.

She maintained an active interest in her subject until the last few weeks of her life, and was present at both the 300th Anniversary celebrations of the foundation of the Royal College of Physicians, Edinburgh, in the summer of 1981, at which she renewed her acquaintance with the Queen, and at the 150th Anniversary of the foundation of the Chair of Pathology in the University of Edinburgh in September, 1981.

The work of Dr. Macgregor will be remembered not only in Glen Lyon but also by generations of students and pathologists throughout the world who will always regard her with both respect and affection.

References

1 Agnes Rose Macgregor (Obituary). Lancet i: 522 (1982).
2 Bain, A.D.; Bowie, J.H.; Flint, W.F.; Beverly, J.K.A.; Beattie, C.P.: Congenital toxoplasmosis simulating haemolytic disease of the newborn. J. Obstet. Gynaec. Br. Emp. 63: 826 (1956).
3 Macgregor, A.R.: Pneumonia in the new-born. Archs Dis. Childh. 14: 323 (1939).
4 Macgregor, A.R.: Tuberculosis in a General Children's Hospital. A pathologist's experience. Edin. med. J. 58: 248 (1951).

5   Macgregor, A.R.; Alexander, W.A.: Pulmonary tuberculosis in children. Edin. med. J. *44:* 561 (1937).
6   Macgregor, A.R.; Green, C.A.: Tuberculosis of the central nervous system with special reference to tuberculous meningitis. J. Path. Bact. *45:* 613 (1937).

D. Bain, MD, Department of Genetic Pathology, Royal Hospital for Sick Children, Edinburgh EH9 1LF (UK)

Perspect. pediatr. Pathol., vol. 11, pp. 6–46 (Karger, Basel 1987)

Pathology of Neonatal Surfactant Deficiency

Bengt Robertson

Departments of Pediatrics and Pathology, St. Göran's Hospital, Stockholm, Sweden

The discovery that the neonatal respiratory distress syndrome (RDS), also known as hyaline membrane disease (HMD), is associated with a deficiency of pulmonary surfactant [1–7] was a major breakthrough in perinatal medicine. It stimulated research teams all over the world to work on basic problems related to the synthesis and release of alveolar surfactant phospholipids in the perinatal period. It also drew attention to the possibilities of preventing or treating RDS by pharmacological means, assisted ventilation, or direct administration of surfactant into the airways. These efforts have resulted in several important new concepts, which have a considerable impact on clinical practice. RDS can be predicted antenatally by analysis of the phospholipid profile in the amniotic fluid [8–13]; glucocorticoids are used to accelerate fetal lung maturation in cases of threatened premature birth [14–20]; application of continuous positive airway pressure (CPAP) has emerged as an effective method for prevention of alveolar collapse in babies with moderate surfactant deficiency [21]; and treatment with exogenous surfactant is gradually being accepted as an alternative to ventilator settings involving dangerously high pressure levels and excessive concentrations of oxygen [22, 23]. The recent rapid development in our understanding of the pathophysiology and clinical management of RDS has been the subject of several extensive reviews [15, 24–27], symposia [28, 29], and a multi-author volume [30].

Although the basic pathogenic mechanisms are well known and therapeutic regimens are available for compensation of neonatal surfactant deficiency, the incidence and mortality of RDS remain unacceptably high, even in developed countries. For instance, the most recent figures for Sweden give an incidence of 0.3% of total births and an overall mortality rate of 24% [31]. The latter disappointing figure is to some extent explained by the association of RDS with prematurity. Patients suffering from RDS are fragile, not only because of their lung problem, but also due to increased susceptibility to infections, inadequate regulation of cerebral blood flow, liability to apneic episodes, hepatic insufficiency, coagulation defects, etc. In spite of highly sophisticated methods for neonatal intensive care, RDS therefore remains a hazardous condition. The disease will probably not be eradicated, and the mortality rate will constitute an important challenge to perinatal medicine as long as preterm deliveries cannot be avoided [32].

However, our increased insight into the underlying pathogenic mechanisms has led to a more rational approach to problems related to assisted ventilation and surfactant replacement in patients with RDS. This, in turn, has reduced the incidence and severity of certain long-term sequelae of the disease, especially bronchopulmonary dysplasia (BPD) [33]. Several important achievements in this field are based on experiences from various RDS models in animals [34]. Experimental work has clarified the pathogenesis of the pulmonary tissue lesions that characterize human RDS [34] and documented the close correlation between the pool sizes of alveolar phospholipids and the severity of clinical symptoms [35, 36]. Well-standardized animal models have also been used for testing potential substitutes for natural surfactant before such preparations were applied in clinical practice [22, 23]. The purpose of this review is to focus on these important links between experimental pathology, human pathology, and clinical perinatal medicine. One particular mission is to emphasize the concept that epithelial necrosis and hyaline membranes are the result of mechanical stress, operating in the surfactant-deficient lung during each ventilatory cycle and therefore iterated several thousand times during the first few hours of extrauterine life.

Physical Properties of Pulmonary Surfactant

Pulmonary surfactant, as defined by its functional characteristics, is a complex of molecules forming a film on the lining layer of alveoli and terminal conducting airways; this film reduces the surface tension of the air-liquid interface, especially on surface compression. Films of pulmonary surfactant exhibit surface tension/surface area hysteresis during cyclic compression, i.e. surface tension at a given surface area is lower at film compression than at film expansion [37–39]. Such films also show rapid spreading; when excess surfactant is applied as a droplet on a hypophase of water, an equilibrium surface tension of 25–30 mN/m (=dynes/cm) is achieved within a second [23] (fig. 1a, b).

These physical properties of the surface film are essential for normal pulmonary function. A low average alveolar surface tension is necessary for postnatal clearance of fluid from the alveoli and later prevents the transudation of fluid from the interstitium. The critical value of alveolar surface tension, above which fetal pulmonary fluid remains unabsorbed or pulmonary edema is likely to occur, depends on the radius of the alveolar curvature [40].

A rapid adsorption of the surface film is also essential during the first breath, when the total air-liquid interface is quickly expanding and surface forces in the terminal bronchioles constitute a major obstacle to lung aeration [41–43]. Once the alveoli have become aerated, they are normally stabilized by the dynamic surface properties of surfactant, mainly by the reduction of the contractile force (referred to as surface tension as long as the surface film is in a fluid state) during surface compression. Another way to describe the same phenomenon is to say that a film of pulmonary surfactant has a low compressibility [44], i.e. it offers a high resistance to compression. A film of surfactant may undergo a phase transition at a certain stage of surface compression due to expulsion of film components, as will be further explained below, and transform from a liquid-crystalline to a solid state. In the compressed, solid state a film of pulmonary surfactant could stabilize alveoli of different size [39, 45].

Perhaps the surface properties during film expansion are also important for normal pulmonary function. Surface tension versus surface area diagrams obtained from films of pulmonary surfactant during cyclic compression characteristically show a wide hysteresis between the compression and expansion parts of the loop (fig. 1b). Applied to alveolar mechanics, this hysteresis means that the airspaces that first expand during the inspiration phase meet a resistance to further inflation due to a rapid and significant increase in alveolar surface tension. They will dilate only when the transpulmonary pressure is further increased and their expansion will then be synchronous with the inflation of a new 'generation' of alveoli. The inflation of these additional airspaces is, in turn, restrained by a rapidly increasing surface tension, throughout the inspiration phase. These surface properties during film expansion would prevent overexpansion of recently inflated alveoli, thus promoting a uniform expansion pat-

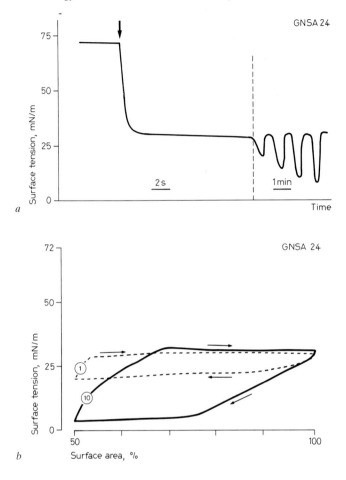

Fig. 1. Surface properties of acetone precipitated fraction of natural surfactant from pig lungs, recorded at 37°C with a modified Wilhelmy balance. *a* Recording of surface tension vs. time after application of 10 µl of surfactant (phospholipid concentration 90 mg/ml) on a hypophase of 0.9% saline with a surface area of 60 cm². Note immediate spreading of the surface film, as indicated by a rapid decrease in surface tension from 72 to about 30 mN/m after surfactant application (arrow). During cycling (right side of the tracing), the surface is compressed by 50%, with a cycling speed of 1/min. There is a gradual decrease in minimal surface tension during the first four cycles. *b* XY recordings from the same experiment, showing the 1st and 10th cycles (additional 10 µl of surfactant were applied to the surface after the 5th cycle). In the 10th cycle, surface tension falls to 6 mN/m already at about 75% surface area. From 75 to 50% surface area there is a plateau in the tracing, corresponding to a squeeze-out of molecules from the surface film.

tern [46]. Another stabilizing factor in the well-inflated lung is 'interdependency'. Since 'the inside of one alveolus is the outside of another' [47], an alveolus localized in an air-expanded area of the lung tends to remain aerated as long as the neighboring airspaces are kept inflated (the same principle also implies that collapse of one alveolus will promote collapse of its neighbor).

Biochemical Characterization of Pulmonary Surfactant

Pulmonary surfactant is a mixture of lipids, mainly phospholipids, synthesized and secreted from the type II alveolar epithelial cells. Its major phospholipid component is dipalmitoylphosphatidylcholine (DPPC). This molecule is the end-product of an enzymatic pathway involving, among other steps, the combination of cytidyldiphosphatecholine with a diglyceride carrying palmitic acid in the alpha-position and an unsaturated fatty acid in the beta-position, and a final deacylation-reacylation process substituting the unsaturated fatty acid chain with a saturated one, usually palmitic acid [48–53].

Surfactant phospholipids are synthesized in the rough endoplasmic reticulum, further processed in the Golgi zone and in the multivesicular bodies [54], and assembled in the type II cells as the characteristic lamellar bodies which contain a relatively larger amount of DPPC than any other known cell organelle or tissue component in the body [55–57]. The surfactant material stored in the lamellar bodies also includes other phosphatidylcholines, 'minor' surfactant phospholipids such as phosphatidylglycerol, phosphatidylethanolamine, and phosphatidylinositol [55–57], apoproteins [54, 58–60], and small amounts of carbohydrates, not yet properly identified [54].

The lamellar bodies are secreted, perhaps in response to beta-adrenergic stimulation of the type II cells [61–62], by simple exocytosis onto the alveolar surface. In the fetus, the secreted lamellar bodies accumulate in the pulmonary fluid. They then join the flux of fetal pulmonary fluid into the amniotic cavity, where they can be demonstrated by conventional electron microscopy [63]. This is the rationale of the principle for determination of fetal lung maturity by analysis of amniotic fluid phospholipids [8–13].

After successful neonatal adaptation, the secreted lamellar bodies enter the liquid lining of the alveoli, where they undergo a series of transformations before their surface active components adsorb to the air-liquid interface. Most probably, the intracellular or newly secreted lamellar body is comparatively 'dry', i.e. it contains a minimum of water molecules between the closely packed phospholipid layers [64]. Using the terminology of Morley et al. [65], the lamellar bodies are packages of 'dry surfactant'. Once secreted into the liquid filling, or lining, the alveolar spaces, the lamellar bodies 'swell', i.e. water accumulates between the lipid bilayers (between the polar heads of the phospholipid molecules) and the surfactant complexes assume the shape of 'tubular myelin'. These structures probably represent a liquid-crystalline phase essential for the subsequent adsorption of the phospholipid molecules to the air-liquid interface [66–73]. The transformation of pulmonary surfactant from lamellar bodies to tubular myelin seems to require the presence of the larger (28,000–36,000 daltons) apoprotein and bivalent cations [74, 75]. Isolated lamellar bodies fail to exhibit in vitro surface properties characteristic of pulmonary surfactant unless calcium ions are added to the system [76].

Electron microscopic studies including observations obtained by freeze-fracture techniques confirm that tubular myelin contains particles other than lipids, most probably a protein component [73, 77]. Film adsorption of surfactant phospholipids is facilitated by the 34,000-dalton [78], the 15,000-dalton [79], and the 5,000-dalton [80] apoproteins, indicating a precise, important role for these proteins in the transformation of surfactant from biophysically inactive lamellar bodies into a highly surface active liquid-crystalline phase.

Under normal conditions, the tubular myelin complexes probably form the major part of the acellular alveolar lining, although its characteristic structure is evident only in sections running parallel or perpendicular to the orientation of the tubules [69]. Transmission electron microscopic studies of the alveolar lining layer after proper fixation demonstrate that the surfactant phospholipid complexes adsorb to the air-liquid interface to form a mono- or frequently multilayered film [67–69, 81, 82]. Freeze-fracture studies of the alveolar surface have confirmed that the alveolar lining layer is continuous and provided additional evidence of crystalline patterns, equivalent to tubular myelin, in the hypophase [83, 84].

Parts of the alveolar surface film are probably lost at each expiration. Compression of the film reduces surface tension below its equilibrium value; as a consequence, the film tends to spread towards the conducting airways [85–87]. A surface film, similar to that in the alveoli, has been demonstrated at bronchiolar level in perfusion-fixed preparations from mammalian lungs [88]. The net movement of this film is directed towards the central airways, not only because of the cyclic variations in alveolar surface tension during respiration, but also due to the action of ciliated cells located between the Clara cells in the bronchiolar mucosa.

With each ventilatory cycle, some molecules in the surface film probably become 'stacked' or lost as stable liposomes to the hypophase (here defined as the liquid layer between the cell border and the surface film), especially following a maximal expiratory effort. Worn-out fragments of the surface film are to some extent ingested by alveolar macrophages [89–91] dwelling in the lining layer. From animal experiments, interaction with surfactant is essential for optimal bactericidal activity of alveolar macrophages [92, 93]. However, uptake by alveolar macrophages represents only a minor pathway for degradation and removal of waste products from the pulmonary surfactant system. From studies on the apparent biological half-life and turnover rate of alveolar phospholipids, about 90% of DPPC and other saturated phosphatidylcholines is recycled [94–97] indicating that the intact molecules are taken up by the alveolar type II cells, reprocessed via the endoplasmic reticulum, Golgi complex and lamellar bodies, and secreted again at the alveolar surface. The precise biochemical mechanisms operating during this recycling process are not known, but the saturated phosphatidylcholines, which have been lost from the surface film, have to be recombined with other molecules to be able to readsorb to the air-liquid interface.

The major component of pulmonary surfactant, DPPC, is a solid at body temperature; its solid-to-liquid-crystal transition temperature is 41.6°C [98]. This implies that DPPC does not spread in an air-liquid interface under normal physiological conditions unless it is mixed with, e.g. unsaturated phosphatidylcholines, phosphatidylglycerol, or phosphatidylinositol. These other phospholipids then serve as 'fluidizers' in the surfactant system, promoting the surface adsorption of DPPC-molecules (via the intermediate tubular-myelin phase). The composition, and therefore the physical state, of the surface film probably changes during the ventilatory cycle. According to this concept, unsaturated phospholipids and other more fluid components become squeezed out of the film during surface compression, leaving the rigid DPPC molecules closely packed in the air-liquid interface. Mixed surfactant phospholipids then rush to the expanding interface during inspiration. However, each expiration again leads to 'refinement' of the surface film, i.e. to increased relative concentration of DPPC molecules. A phase transition from liquid-crystalline to solid state at a certain stage of film compression then annihilates the destabilizing effect of surface tension in a system of alveoli of different size [39, 45, 99].

The concept of a cyclic molecular rearrangement in the alveolar air-liquid interface during ventilation thus solves the paradox that a film of pulmonary surfactant at 37°C is characterized by two physical properties which seem to be mutually exclusive: high fluidity allowing rapid adsorption and high rigidity offering effective resistance to surface compression. Neonatal RDS reflects a disturbance of these delicate mechanisms, caused by deficient supply of surfactant phospholipids in the alveolar spaces [1–7], or inactivation of these molecules by 'surfactant inhibitors' [100].

Pathophysiology of RDS in Relation to Alveolar Surface Properties

Some important consequences of neonatal surfactant deficiency are easily understood from the principles outlined above. Pioneering investigations were made by Gruenwald and co-workers [101–106] who, working on autopsy material from newborn infants, demonstrated that pressure-volume recordings from lungs with HMD are characterized by abnormally high opening pressure and poor stability on deflation.

Direct microscopic observations of the lung surface during a simulated first breath confirms that the pressure gradient required to 'push' the air-liquid interface through the terminal bronchiole is significantly higher in immature experimental animals than in mature ones [107–110]. Even at a static inflation pressure of 35 cm H_2O, the pattern of alveolar expansion is irregular in immature rabbits, whereas a uniform expansion is obtained in mature animals at a pressure of only 25 cm H_2O [108]. The same experimental model also shows a striking difference between immature and mature lungs when transpulmonary pressure is reduced to 0 cm H_2O after maximal inflation. Virtually all alveoli of the immature lung 'collapse', i.e. return to the fetal fluid-filled state, whereas the alveoli of the mature animal remain aerated (fig. 2).

That these variations in mechanical behaviour reflect differences in the supply of alveolar surfactant is perhaps best shown by the conversion of the physical properties of an immature lung into those of a mature lung, simply by depositing an adequate amount of natural pulmonary surfactant in the tracheal fluid [43, 107, 108].

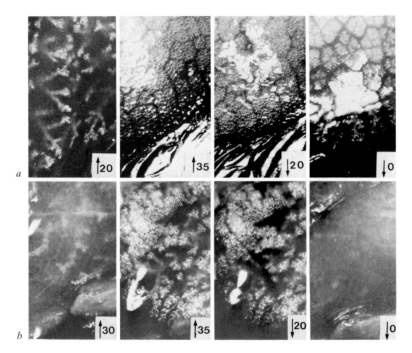

Fig. 2. Alveolar expansion patterns in neonatal rabbit lungs, documented by direct observation of the pleural surface in a dissection microscope (×10). The photographs were obtained during pressure-volume recordings simulating a first breath. Insufflation (↑) and deflation (↓) pressure levels are given in cm H_2O in the right lower corner of each photograph. Upper panel (*a*): Nearly full-term lung (gestational age 30 days) showing incipient alveolar expansion at insufflation pressure 20 cm H_2O and uniform expansion at pressure 35 cm H_2O. The pattern remains uniform during deflation and the alveoli are still aerated when pressure is lowered to 0 cm H_2O. Lower panel (*b*): Premature lung (gestational age 28 days) showing virtually no alveolar expansion at inflation pressure 30 cm H_2O, and incomplete expansion even at pressure 35 cm H_2O. In this surfactant-deficient lung, the alveoli return to the fluid-filled state at the end of deflation. Reprinted with permission from Grossmann [108].

This latter observation suggested to us [43] that neonatal RDS might be prevented, or treated, by surfactant replacement via the airways, a contention today supported by several independent investigators [23].

The classical symptoms and signs of RDS – tachypnea, grunting, intercostal and sternal retractions, cyanosis, failure to establish an adequate functional residual capacity, and reduced dynamic lung compliance [25–

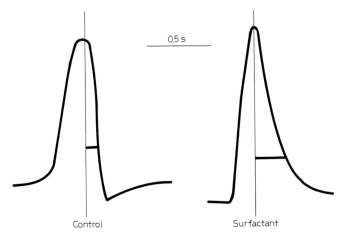

0.5 s

Control   Surfactant

Fig. 3. Volume tracings from immature newborn rabbit lungs, obtained during artificial ventilation with standardized tidal volume (10 ml/kg). The animals were delivered on day 27 of gestation. The left tracing is from a control animal, the right from a littermate, treated with natural surfactant via the tracheal cannula before onset of ventilation. Note that the expiration phase is prolonged in the surfactant-treated animal because the alveolar surface film of phospholipid molecules offers a significant resistance to surface compression. Time constant of expiration is indicated by horizontal bar in each tracing.

27, 111–116] – can all be attributed to the disturbance of alveolar mechanics described above, and hence to the underlying surfactant deficiency. The chest wall retractions reflect the combination of 'stiff lungs' and 'soft thorax', characteristic of immature babies, together with the need for a high transpulmonary pressure to overcome surface forces in terminal bronchioles during inspiration. The liability of the alveoli to collapse at end-expiration is reflected by low functional residual capacity, right-to-left shunting through nonventilated portions of the lungs, and by the miliary 'reticulogranular' type of atelectasis documented radiologically [27].

The time constant of the expiration phase is reduced in lungs with surfactant deficiency; volume tracings from immature experimental animals show that air is rapidly 'ejaculated' during the expiration phase, whereas in mature animals the expulsion of air is a much slower process, modulated by surfactant molecules solidifying in the air-liquid interface during surface compression [117, 118]. As in static pressure-volume recordings, the in vivo physical properties of the immature lung can be transformed into a mature pattern by surfactant replacement via the airways [118, 119] (fig. 3).

During spontaneous ventilation, the surfactant-deficient baby tries to prevent alveolar collapse by increasing the respiratory frequency or, more importantly, by grunting. During the latter maneuver the baby nearly closes the glottis, thereby increasing the expiratory airway resistance [120, 121]. Grunting results in a period of low, nearly constant flow during the first part of expiration, and a positive transpulmonary pressure gradient associated with a prominent peak of flow at end expiration [115, 116]. This compensatory mechanism is obviously not available to intubated patients who may depend on certain therapeutic regimens (application of CPAP or surfactant replacement) for maintenance of alveolar stability.

Epithelial Lesions Associated with Surfactant Deficiency

The alveolar epithelial cells are linked by 'tight junctions', a system of ridges and strands on the lateral cell surfaces [122, 123]. A measure of the permeability of these junctions is the 'pore equivalent radius', which for the nondistended neonatal alveolar epithelium is in the order of 0.6 nm. When this figure is related to the corresponding value for the alveolar capillary endothelium, 10–15 nm, and to the diffusion radius of an albumin molecule, 3.4 nm, it follows that the intact alveolar epithelium – in contrast to the capillary endothelium – is impermeable to protein [124]. Another implication is that the appearance of protein in the alveolar spaces is the result of pollution with exogenous material, active secretion (as in the case of immunoglobulins or surfactant apoproteins) or breakdown of the epithelial barrier. In lambs with RDS, the epithelium of peripheral airspaces is characterized by an increased permeability to protein [35, 125], a leakage which is best explained by disruption of tight junctions and necrosis of epithelial cells [124].

A histologic section from a surfactant-deficient lung shows only collapsed, or fluid-filled alveoli, since the alveolar air-liquid interfaces return to the bronchioles at end-expiration (fig. 2). It is perhaps less obvious that surfactant deficiency could induce necrosis of bronchiolar and alveolar epithelium. However, such a damage can be interpreted as the result of shear forces on the epithelium, secondary to overdistension of bronchioles proximal to a level where, during the inspiration phase, the air-liquid interface tends to be arrested by surface tension [126]. The shear forces

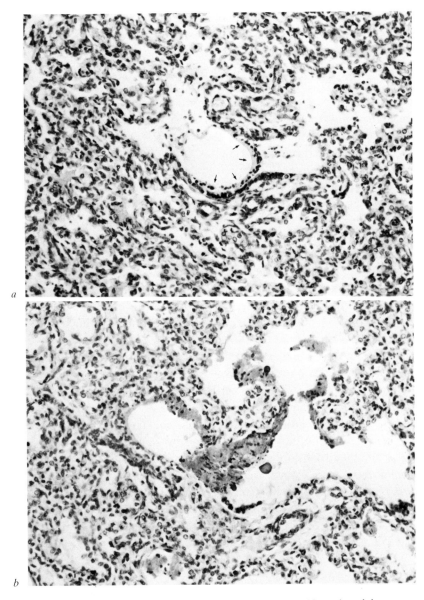

Fig. 4. Early stage of HMD in premature twins. HE ×220. *a* Necrosis and desquamation of bronchiolar epithelium (arrows) in twin I (1,050 g). This patient died from respiratory insufficiency shortly after birth, in spite of resuscitation efforts. *b* Lung section from twin II (1,070 g), showing typical hyaline membranes in bronchioles and alveoli. This baby died at the age of 5.5 h.

might also damage the alveolar epithelium since the expansion pattern of a surfactant-deficient lung is asynchronous and therefore irregular throughout the ventilatory cycle.

That epithelial lesions characteristically first affect the terminal bronchioles [127–130] can be concluded from observations in immature twins dying from RDS at different intervals after birth [131]. Necrosis and desquamation of bronchiolar epithelium occur in the surfactant-deficient infant within a few minutes after birth, even if the baby has only been gasping without assisted ventilation [132] (fig. 4a). This observation might have forensic implications as the presence of such lesions in an otherwise nonaerated parenchyma establishes attempts to expand the lungs either by spontaneous efforts or artificial means. At a later stage, the necrotic bronchiolar epithelial cells coalesce to form the well-known hyaline membranes (fig. 4b), and the necrotizing lesions usually spread to involve part of the alveolar epithelium as well [133–139] (fig. 5).

Considering the pathogenesis of the hyaline membranes, it is to be expected that these eosinophilic 'red herrings' [140] contain cellular debris [133–135, 137–139], Feulgen-positive material including nucleoproteins [141], fibrin [133, 139, 142] and other large molecules leaking from the denuded epithelial surfaces. Leakage of bilirubin into the airspaces may result in 'yellow hyaline membranes' [143]. The membranes are more prominent in infants dying from RDS after 2–3 days of illness than in those dying within the first 24 h after birth [144] and may eventually form plugs obstructing the terminal airways [145].

Although the epithelial lesions should not change with the time interval between death and sampling (except for structural alterations due to autolysis) the expansion pattern of the lungs seems to depend on this particular time factor. Lauweryns [137] reported that alveolar atelectasis was less prominent in samples fixed by immersion in formalin shortly after death than in specimens obtained from the same lungs at a later interval. This suggests a postmortem centripetal movement of the air-liquid interfaces due to the absence of a stabilizing film of surfactant phospholipids.

Similarly, lung sections from surfactant-deficient premature newborn animals show nonaerated alveoli after immersion-fixation, even if the trachea is clamped at end-inspiration after ventilation with a pressure which should have caused significant expansion of the alveolar compartment [146]. The conclusion from these data is that the lungs are best fixed by vascular perfusion, preferably while the parenchyma is kept inflated with a known transpulmonary pressure. Only then will the histologic sec-

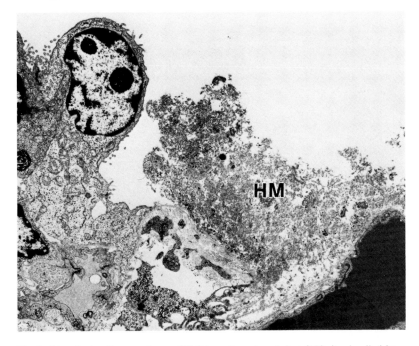

Fig. 5. Alveolar hyaline membrane (HM) in an immature infant (830 g), who died from RDS at the age of 9.5 h. Material for electron microscopy was obtained at autopsy within 1 h after death. The membrane contains cellular debris, representing remnants of necrotic epithelium. ×4,100. Electron microphotograph provided courtesy of Dr. Ernest Cutz, Toronto.

tions show a configuration of alveoli which is representative of the prefixation state.

Pulmonary Vasculature in RDS

Neonatal RDS has been considered the result of 'pulmonary ischemia' [112] or 'pulmonary hypoperfusion' [147, 148] associated with right-to-left shunting through a widely patent ductus arteriosus, especially during the early stage of the disease [25, 27, 149]. This concept disregarded the considerable proportion of shunting through nonventilated areas of the lung parenchyma [26, 150, 151].

Some morphologic support for the 'hypoperfusion theory' was provided by Lauweryns and co-workers [152, 153], who reported poor end-arterial and capillary filling in postmortem pulmonary angiograms from

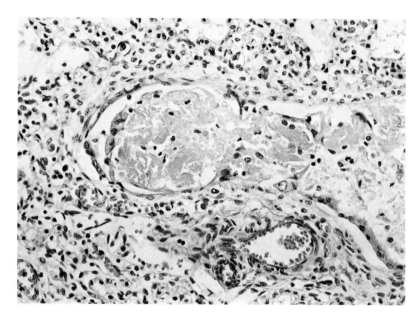

Fig. 6. Organizing HMD in a premature infant (1,330 g), who died from RDS at the age of 11 days. The patient was treated with artificial ventilation since shortly after birth, requiring high pressure levels (up to 50 cm H_2O) and periods of 100% oxygen. This bronchiole contains fragmented hyaline material, infiltrated by inflammatory cells and undermined by regenerating epithelium. HE. ×220.

infants with RDS. However, these results were not confirmed in a more recent microangiographic study [154], in which the pulmonary vascular pattern of infants with RDS did not differ from that of patients dying from other diseases in the neonatal period. Morphometric studies of the pulmonary arteries in RDS have given conflicting data as to the presence of medial hypertrophy or vasoconstriction [155, 156]. Today, the idea that pulmonary hypoperfusion would be a triggering factor in RDS seems obsolete, especially as pulmonary vasoconstriction with right-to-left shunting through a patent ductus arteriosus is a nonspecific reaction to arterial hypoxemia in newborn infants.

Lauweryns and co-workers [157, 158] emphasized that the lymphatics are usually dilated in lungs from patients with HMD. It is not likely that this dilatation is an expression of increased lymph flow. Data from experiments on newborn lambs indicate that immature animals with surfactant deficiency have a lower pulmonary lymph flow than full-term lambs [159,

160], probably reflecting delayed resorption of fluid from the airspaces. Dilatation of lymphatics in RDS might be secondary to abnormally high retractive forces in the air-liquid interfaces of the lungs leading to increased negative interstitial pressure and favoring the accumulation of fluid in septal tissue and lymphatics.

'Organizing' HMD; Bronchopulmonary Dysplasia (BPD)

In survivors of RDS, the hyaline membranes fragment and resorb (fig. 6). This repair phase, sometimes referred to as 'organizing HMD', lasts from the 4th or the 5th day of life until the age of about 2 weeks [130, 136, 137, 144, 161–163]. In severely ill infants dependent on artificial ventilation, the repair phase merges with the early stage of BPD [130, 164–174].

Organizing HMD is also characterized by interstitial proliferation of fibroblasts and histiocytes, and an increasing number of macrophages in the alveolar spaces [130, 136, 137, 144, 161–163]. The hyaline membranes become undermined by the regenerating epithelium and eventually engulfed by the alveolar macrophages. The number of lamellar bodies in type II cells, reduced during the early stage of HMD [130, 136, 175, 176] increases [130, 176] and normal surface activity can be demonstrated in lung extracts from infants surviving the first few days [130, 136]. These morphologic observations are based on autopsy specimens from patients dying in spite of intensive care, usually involving respirator treatment. Therefore they do not necessarily represent the natural course of the disease, but rather an evolution compromised by epithelial lesions due to oxygen toxicity and high-pressure ventilation.

BPD is a chronic neonatal lung disease, iatrogenic in the sense that it is induced by artificial ventilation. The underlying condition necessitating respirator treatment is usually HMD, although cases of BPD have also been reported in patients with recurrent apnea subjected to artificial ventilation [177, 178] (fig. 7b). The clinical manifestations are persistent oxygen dependency, tachypnea, reduction of lung compliance and increased airway resistance, a radiologic pattern of interstitial infiltrates and focal hyperexpansion of the lung parenchyma, and evidence of right ventricular hypertrophy. The gross and histologic findings at autopsy in typical cases include an irregular alveolar expansion pattern with areas of hyperdistension alternating with areas of atelectasis. A recent morphometric study showed

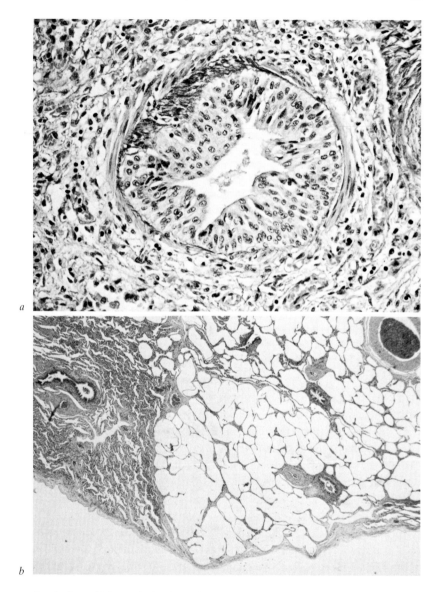

Fig. 7. Bronchiolar and alveolar lesions in BPD. *a* Regenerating airway epithelium showing hyperplasia and early squamous cell metaplasia. This premature infant (birth weight 970 g) developed symptoms of apnea and RDS shortly after birth, necessitating artificial ventilation with insufflation pressure >30 cm H_2O and periods of 100% oxygen. The patient remained dependent on the respirator and died at the age of 3.5 months. In both lungs there were areas of emphysema alternating with atelectasis, interstitial fibrosis, and hypertrophy of

a striking reduction of both alveolar number and total alveolar surface area in an infant dying from BPD at the age of 33 months [179], suggesting that in this disease, the postnatal growth of the terminal airspaces is not associated with normal alveolar multiplication. There is also interstitial fibroplasia (especially in cases developing from organizing HMD) with excessive deposition of collagen in alveolar and interlobular septa, particularly in less well-expanded areas. Other characteristic findings are hyperplasia or squamous metaplasia of regenerating airway epithelium (fig. 7a), medial hypertrophy in muscular pulmonary arteries indicating pulmonary hypertension [33, 130, 164–174], and increased number of neuroendocrine cells in the bronchiolar mucosa [180].

In a recent retrospective study of 18 autopsy cases representing various stages of clinically verified BPD, we found squamous metaplasia of bronchiolar epithelium only in infants ventilated with comparatively high pressure ($\leq$50 cm H_2O) until the final stage of the disease, and emphysema (arbitrarily defined as alveolar diameter $\geq$300 μm, irrespective of whether this enlargement is caused by destruction of parenchyma or by growth without adequate alveolar multiplication) only in infants over 1 month of age. We also found that the irregular expansion pattern, with areas of atelectasis alternating with emphysema, might persist for several months after the end of the ventilator treatment (fig. 7b). We concluded from these observations that, in BPD, the alveolar lesions are less readily reversible than those affecting the airway mucosa [181].

Although BPD was originally interpreted as the result of pulmonary oxygen toxicity [33, 166, 173], retrospective studies of large autopsy series have indicated that the severity of airway lesions is more correlated to the peak pressure levels used during artificial ventilation than to the accumulated dose of oxygen [130, 182, 183]. However, the role of oxygen toxicity

---

muscular pulmonary arteries. The epithelial lesion shown in the microphotograph can be documented by cytologic examination of tracheal effluent (cf. fig. 8b). Hematoxylin, Weigert, van Gieson. ×230. *b* Late stage of BPD in an infant (birth weight 1,400 g) dying at the age of 9 months with cor pulmonale. The patient was treated with artificial ventilation for recurrent apneic episodes in the neonatal period and was not weaned from the respirator until the age of 2 months. Insufflation pressure and oxygen levels ranged up to 30 cm H_2O and 45%, respectively. This histologic section shows a persistent, mosaic-like pattern with areas of hyperexpansion alternating with areas of atelectasis. The mucosa of the bronchioles, however, is normal. This picture is not easily distinguished from that seen in the Wilson-Mikity syndrome. HE. ×23.

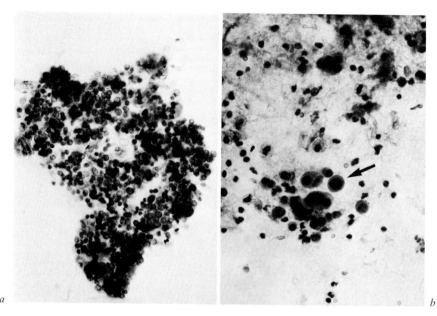

Fig. 8. Cytologic features of neonatal airway epithelial lesions induced by artificial ventilation. The samples were obtained by gentle, routine rinsing of the bronchial tree. Papanicolaou stain. *a* Desquamated sheet of columnar respiratory cells without evidence of squamous metaplasia in patient with persistent fetal circulation; age 2 days (Merritt, grade I). ×210. *b* Transitional metaplastic cells (arrow) and moderate, nonspecific inflammatory reaction in infant with RDS; age 6 days (Merritt, grade III). ×340.

can certainly not be excluded; this holds particularly for the interstitial fibroplasia, one of the characteristic features of the disease. The etiology of BPD is probably multifactorial [184] and well summarized by the words 'oxygen plus pressure plus time' [185].

BPD versus Wilson-Mikity Syndrome

Morphologically, BPD has several features in common with the Wilson-Mikity syndrome [186–190]. Both diseases have similar radiologic appearance and are characterized histologically by emphysema and atelectasis in a mosaic pattern, irregular fibrosis, and medial hypertrophy in muscular pulmonary arteries. However, whereas epithelial hyperplasia and squamous metaplasia are typical findings in the airways in the subacute phase of BPD, they are absent in the Wilson-Mikity syndrome [187,

188]. Clinically, infants with the Wilson-Mikity syndrome usually have no respiratory symptoms in the immediate neonatal period [189], whereas most cases of BPD are secondary to acute lung disorders developing shortly after birth.

The labelling of these two chronic neonatal lung disorders is complicated by a phase of severe respiratory insufficiency in some infants with the Wilson-Mikity syndrome, necessitating artificial ventilation. Lesions in the airway mucosa similar to those in BPD might then appear, and a morphologic differential diagnosis between the diseases is, therefore, not always possible.

Cytologic Diagnosis of BPD

The epithelial lesions of BPD can be detected at an early stage by cytologic examination of material obtained by gentle tracheal lavage [191–193]. Since rinsing of the tracheal tube and larger airways is, in most units, part of the routine of respirator treatment, sampling for this type of cytologic examination does not add extra burden on the patients.

The various cytologic abnormalities in tracheal aspirates from RDS-patients on artificial ventilation include sheets of desquamated, but otherwise intact ciliated epithelium (grade I), and various forms of transition from respiratory columnar to squamous metaplastic cells with granular chromatin and prominent chromocenters (grade II-III) (fig. 8). This grading system was proposed by Merritt et al. [191, 192], who noted that only cytologic changes classified as grade III were associated with the development of BPD. As another significant observation, squamous metaplasia appears in cytologic samples several days before BPD can be verified radiologically. This new diagnostic tool can identify patients-at-risk in whom every possible effort should be made to define a ventilator setting that avoids further damage to the pulmonary parenchyma.

Experimental RDS in Rabbits

The rabbit has a normal gestational period of 31 days. The lungs of a rabbit fetus delivered on day 27 are similar to those of a human fetus of about 25 weeks' gestation, i.e. the structure of the alveolar epithelium is compatible with gas exchange, but adequate amounts of surfactant phospholipids have not yet accumulated in the pulmonary fluid [194–197]. As in man [198–201], the timetable of fetal lung maturation has a notable sex difference, favoring the females [202, 203]. Immature rabbits are unable to generate the transpulmonary pressure gradient necessary to move the air-liquid interfaces through terminal bronchioles and, therefore, die from respiratory insufficiency shortly after birth [204]. These animals do not seem to try hard to survive; they usually give up after gasping for a few minutes without exhibiting the tenacious respiratory efforts that are characteristic of a human infant with surfactant deficiency. Immature rabbits have to be kept on artificial ventilation to remain alive beyond the immediate neonatal period.

Ventilating these surfactant-deficient animals is impossible without causing considerable damage to the bronchiolar epithelium; after only a few minutes of artificial [205], or spontaneous [206] ventilation, necrotic and desquamating cells can be observed in bronchioles and alveoli (fig. 9a, b). If the period of ventilation is prolonged to 15–30 min or more, these degenerating cells coalesce to form hyaline membranes similar to those seen in immature infants dying from neonatal RDS [118, 119, 205] (fig. 10). The premature rabbit fetus is a useful model of neonatal RDS, especially as there is a good correlation between the amount of surfactant phospholipids in the alveolar spaces [194–197], the mechanical properties of the lungs [107–110, 117, 207] and the liability to develop morphologic evidence of HMD during artificial ventilation [117, 118].

Studies in our laboratory have shown that the in vivo compliance of the immature rabbit lungs can be improved, and the development of epithelial lesions prevented, by administration of natural surfactant into the airways before the onset of artificial ventilation [119]. This effect was observed even if the surfactant-treated animals were grossly overventilated with a standardized high insufflation pressure [208]. Treatment with natural surfactant also results in a striking improvement of alveolar expansion in histologic sections [119, 208–210] (fig. 12) and reduces the leakage of protein into the airspaces [211].

To analyze to what extent treatment with surfactant was effective in immature animals in whom epithelial lesions had already developed, Nilsson et al. [212] treated premature newborn rabbits with surfactant *after* a 10-min period of artificial ventilation, and then at 30-min intervals until no further improvement of lung-thorax mechanics was observed. The dose of surfactant required for a therapeutic response was higher than in experiments involving surfactant replacement at birth [119, 208] but two

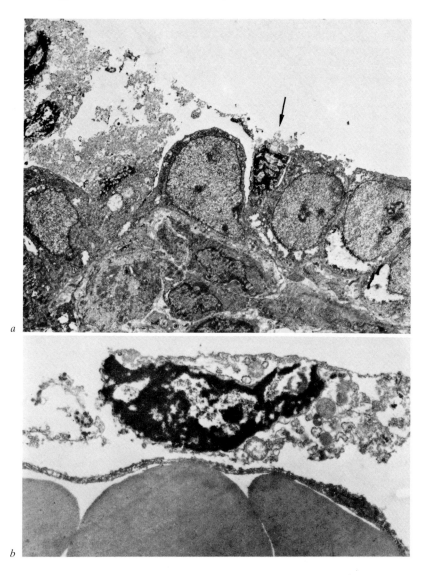

Fig. 9. Electron microphotographs showing early epithelial lesions in surfactant-deficient, immature newborn rabbits, delivered on day 27 of gestation and ventilated for 5 min with insufflation pressure 35 cm H$_2$O. The development of these lesions can be prevented by tracheal administration of surfactant before onset of ventilation [119, 208]. *a* Necrosis of bronchiolar epithelium (arrow, and upper left) representing an early stage of HMD. ×3,800. *b* Similar lesion at alveolar level. The field shows a bulging alveolar capillary coated by necrotic, disintegrating epithelium. ×10,100.

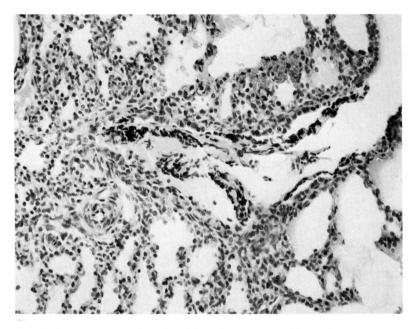

Fig. 10. Conspicuous necrosis and shedding of bronchiolar epithelium in surfactant-deficient newborn rabbit; gestational age 27 days. This animal was ventilated for 60 min with standardized tidal volume (10 ml/kg). The epithelial lesions, similar to those in figure 4a, are probably caused by abnormal shear forces in the bronchiolar mucosa. HE. ×230.

instillations of surfactant (each dose = about 13 mg phospholipids/kg) usually resulted in significant enhancement of lung-thorax compliance. Treatment with surfactant also seemed to arrest the development of bronchiolar epithelial lesions at a stage corresponding to that seen in most immature animals after about 10 min of artificial ventilation, although some of these experimental animals were ventilated for more than two hours. As in earlier experiments [119, 208–210], lung sections from surfactant-treated animals showed significantly improved alveolar expansion. These observations clearly indicate that surfactant replacement is effective when the treatment is given during the early course of experimental HMD.

Surfactant-deficient newborn rabbits also benefit from artificial ventilation with prolonged inspiration phase, at least in the frequency range 20–60 min [213]. These data from animal experiments agree with earlier clinical observations in patients with RDS reported by Reynolds and coworkers [214–216]. Surfactant-deficient neonatal lungs usually collapse at

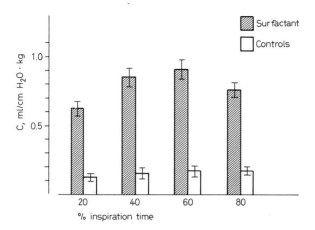

Fig. 11. Lung-thorax compliance (C) in artificially ventilated immature newborn rabbits; gestational age 27 days. The animals were ventilated with pressure 25 cm H_2O, frequency 40/min, and inspiration time varying from 20 to 80%. Half of the animals were treated with natural surfactant before the onset of ventilation. Compliance is markedly increased in surfactant-treated animals (p vs. controls <0.001 for all ventilator settings), but the optimal effect is obtained at 40–60% inspiration time (p 40 vs. 20% <0.01). Based on data from Lachmann et al. [219].

end-expiration, i.e. the alveoli tend to become refilled with unresorbed fetal pulmonary fluid (fig. 2). This implies that not only surface tension, but also viscosity of pulmonary fluid offers a resistance to aeration during the inspiration phase [217, 218]. Therefore, inspiratory efforts will result in alveolar expansion only if the transpulmonary pressure gradient is high enough to overcome surface tension in the finer conducting airways *and* if this pressure is maintained long enough to allow for displacement of fluid from the airways. A beneficial effect can also be obtained by shortening the expiration phase until the (time-dependent) collapse of the surfactant-deficient alveoli is prevented [213].

In recent similar experiments reported by Lachmann et al. [219], the protocol included a combination of surfactant replacement and variation of the inspiration-expiration ratio at a standardized respiratory frequency, 40/min. Treatment with surfactant resulted in significant improvement of both lung-thorax compliance (fig. 11) and alveolar air expansion (fig. 12). The latter effect was documented by conventional morphometric technique [219] as well as by automated image analysis, a useful method for evaluation of expansion patterns in the neonatal lung [220]. Alveolar ex-

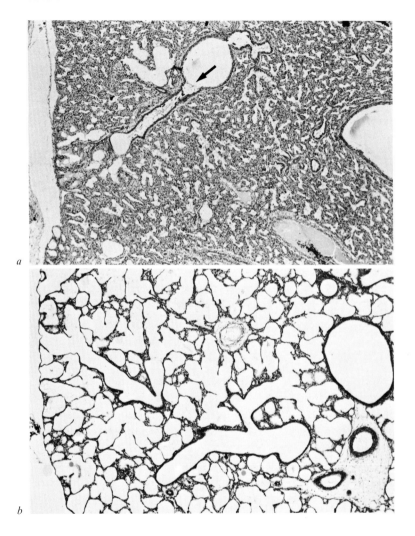

Fig. 12. Effect of surfactant replacement on alveolar expansion pattern in immature newborn rabbits; gestational age 27 days. These sections were obtained from animals ventilated with pressure 25 cm H$_2$O, frequency 40/min, and 80% inspiration time. The lungs were fixed by immersion in formalin after clamping of the trachea at end-inspiration. HE. ×45. *a* Control animal showing virtually nonaerated parenchyma with necrosis and desquamation of bronchiolar epithelium (arrow). *b* Surfactant-treated animal with regular pattern of well-aerated alveoli and no epithelial lesions. From Lachmann et al. [219], reprinted with permission.

pansion was more uniform in surfactant-treated animals ventilated with 60–80% inspiration time than in those ventilated with 20–40%, indicating that prolonged inspiration resulted in increased recruitment of aerated alveoli. In this experimental model, neonatal surfactant deficiency seems best compensated for by a combination of surfactant replacement and optimal ventilator setting.

Since the rabbit has a comparatively short gestational period and regularly produces litters with multiple fetuses, the rabbit RDS model is most suitable for testing of pharmacological methods for acceleration of fetal lung maturation [221, 222] and for evaluation of potential surfactant substitutes [223].

The surfactant preparations so far tested in the rabbit model include Fujiwara's mixture of bovine natural surfactant and synthetic lipids [224–226], emulsified synthetic surfactant [227], dry artificial surfactant containing only DPPC and phosphatidylglycerol [45, 228], protein-depleted surfactant prepared according to Berggren et al. [229], and surfactant purified from human amniotic fluid [230]. The common aim of all these investigators was to produce a surfactant preparation for treatment, or prophylaxis, of neonatal RDS. Several of these surfactant substitutes have later been used in clinical trials, in general with very promising results [231–234].

Experimental RDS in Lambs and Monkeys

RDS models based on prematurely delivered fetuses from larger animals, such as sheep and monkeys, have at least one obvious advantage in comparison with the rabbit model: samples for determination of blood gases can easily be obtained. The setting of the ventilator system can thus be adjusted with respect to the same parameters as those used for monitoring human patients in the corresponding clinical situation. Studies on artificially ventilated preterm lambs have confirmed the beneficial effect of surfactant replacement on lung mechanics and lung morphology, earlier documented in rabbits, and added the important observation that blood gases are significantly improved following surfactant replacement [235–240].

Similar experiments have documented the inverse correlation between the pool size of alveolar phosphatidylcholine and the severity of neonatal respiratory insufficiency [35, 36], and showed that lambs with surfactant deficiency have a substantial bidirectional flux of protein across the alveolar epithelium [35, 125, 241]. This leakage of protein can be significantly reduced by administration of natural surfactant either at birth or during a later stage of neonatal adaptation [125], probably because this treatment prevents or arrests the development of epithelial damage [119, 208, 212].

One of the proteins leaking into the airways of immature lungs in lambs seems to be a potent inhibitor of pulmonary surfactant [125, 238, 242, 243]. This particular protein, which has a molecular weight of 110,000 daltons [243], has been identified also in tracheal effluents from babies with RDS [100, 244]. Surfactant inhibitors leaking into the terminal airspaces via the damaged epithelium would tend to aggravate the course of the disease, interfere with the natural recovery phase, and reduce the therapeutic effect of exogenous surfactant. Perhaps our original concept is still valid: surfactant replacement should be most effective when the treatment is given prophylactically at birth, before epithelial lesions have developed in the lungs [43].

Enhörning et al. [245] studied lung function in immature newborn rhesus monkeys, in which surfactant was instilled into the airways before the first breath. The results were similar to those obtained in the lamb experiments [235–240]; treatment with surfactant resulted in improvement of blood gas values and in prolonged survival. Combined light and electron microscopic studies on the same lungs were reported separately by Cutz et al. [246]. Since the period of artificial ventilation ranged between 4.5 and 6 h, control animals showed abundant epithelial lesions including hyaline membranes in both bronchioles and alveoli. As expected, surfactant-treated monkeys had clearly improved aeration of the alveolar compartment, but the expansion pattern was not quite uniform. Some areas of collapsed alveoli were found also in the treated animals, suggesting that the dose of surfactant was suboptimal or that it had not spread to all parts of the lungs. These collapsed areas exhibited epithelial lesions similar to those found throughout the lungs of control animals. This observation fits our concept that epithelial lesions in surfactant-deficient lungs are caused by abnormal shear forces in the pulmonary parenchyma [126, 208]. The basic problem in HMD is that the alveoli have to be 'ripped open' with each inspiration.

Recent studies on immature newborn monkeys have revealed a correlation between deficiency of alveolar macrophages and severity of RDS [247]. This new observation raises the possibility that treatment with exogenous surfactant might accelerate recovery from RDS by recruitment of alveolar macrophages. These macrophages have an important mission during organizing HMD by digesting and removing membranes and cell debris from the airspaces [130, 136, 137, 144, 161–163]. In the mammalian fetus, the influx of macrophages into the alveolar spaces starts shortly before term [90], perhaps as the result of chemotaxis exerted by the accumulating surfactant phospholipids [248]. The antibacterial defense system of the lung seems to depend on a proper interaction between alveolar macrophages and surfactant phospholipids [92, 93] and failure of this mechanism could explain why, in some patients with surfactant deficiency, the symptoms of RDS are apparently overshadowed by complications due to severe pulmonary infection developing shortly after birth [249].

Concluding Remarks

Reflecting the bias of the author, this article has focused on problems related to alveolar surface physics and experimental models of RDS. The reason for choosing this perspective is that research in these particular areas has significantly increased the understanding of the pathology of neonatal RDS and recently resulted in a new therapeutic approach: surfactant replacement [23, 250, 251]. The beneficial effect of this treatment has now been documented both in animal experiments and in clinical trials. The first 10 patients reported by Fujiwara et al. [231] showed a dramatic improvement of blood gas values and of radiologic changes after a single dose of 'artificial surfactant' via the airways. Similar results were obtained by other investigators [232, 234, 252–254] in more recent clinical trials. The results are impressive, especially as these were severely ill patients, dependent on artificial ventilation. They were treated at a stage when widespread epithelial damage must already have developed in the pulmonary parenchyma. Although treatment with surfactant did not repair these lesions immediately, it facilitated gas exchange during the recovery phase and probably reduced the risk of BPD.

Fujiwara's first clinical trial provides the link in a series of key observations on the pathogenesis of neonatal RDS. It was the logical application of knowledge that infants with RDS suffer from surfactant deficiency [1] and of data from numerous animal experiments documenting that this deficiency can be compensated for by surfactant replacement [22]. It reminds us that experimental pathology still constitutes a sound basis for clinical medicine.

Acknowledgements

This work was supported by the Swedish Medical Research Council (project No. 3351), The Swedish National Association against Heart and Chest Diseases, The 'Expressen' Prenatal Research Foundation, The Research Funds of the Karolinska Institute, Allmänna Barnbördshusets Minnesfond, and Stiftelsen Samariten.
Dr. Magnus Nasiell kindly reviewed the section on cytological diagnosis of bronchopulmonary dysplasia.

References

1   Avery, M.E.; Mead, J.: Surface properties in relation to atelectasis and hyaline membrane disease. Am. J. Dis. Child. *97:* 517 (1959).

2   Reynolds, E.O.R.; Orzalesi, M.M.; Motoyama, E.K.; et al.: Surface properties of saline extracts from lungs of newborn infants. Acta. paediat. scand. *54:* 511 (1965).

3   Brumley, G.W.; Hodson, W.A.; Avery, M.E.: Lung phospholipids and surface tension correlations in infants with and without hyaline membrane disease and in adults. Pediatrics, Springfield *40:* 13 (1967).

4   Gandy, G.; Bradbrooke, J.G.; Naidoo, B.T.; et al.: Comparison of methods for evaluating surface properties of lung in perinatal period. Archs Dis. Childh. *43:* 8 (1968).

5   Reynolds, E.O.R.; Roberton, N.R.C.; Wigglesworth, J.S.: Hyaline membrane disease, respiratory distress, and surfactant deficiency. Pediatrics, Springfield *42:* 758 (1968).

6   Adams, F.H.; Fujiwara, T.; Emmanouilides, G.C.; et al.: Lung phospholipids of human fetuses and infants with and without hyaline membrane disease. J. Pediat. *77:* 833 (1970).

7   Boughton, K.; Gandy, G.; Gairdner, D.: Hyaline membrane disease. II. Lung lecithin. Archs Dis. Childh. *45:* 311 (1970).

8   Gluck, L.; Kulovich, M.V.; Borer, R.C., Jr.; et al.: Diagnosis of the respiratory distress syndrome by amniocentesis. Am. J. Obstet. Gynec. *109:* 440 (1971).

9   Ekelund, L.; Arvidson, G.; Åstedt, B.: Amniotic fluid lecithin and its fatty acid composition in respiratory distress syndrome. J. Obstet. Gynaec. Br. Commonw. *80:* 912 (1973).

10 Hallman, M.; Kulovich, M.; Kirkpatrick, E.; et al.: Phosphatidylinositol and phosphatidylglycerol in amniotic fluid. Indices of lung maturity. Am. J. Obstet. Gynec. *125:* 613 (1976).

11 Torday, J.; Carson, L.; Lawson, E.E.: Saturated phosphatidylcholine in amniotic fluid and prediction of the respiratory distress syndrome. New Engl. J. Med. *301:* 1013 (1979).

12 Kulovich, M.V.; Hallman, M.; Gluck, L.: The lung profile. I. Normal pregnancy. Am. J. Obstet. Gynec. *135:* 57 (1979).

13 Kulovich, M.V.; Gluck, L.: The lung profile II. Complicated pregnancy. Am. J. Obstet. Gynec. *135:* 64 (1979).

14 Liggins, G.C.; Howie, R.N.: A controlled trial of antepartum glucocorticoid treatment for prevention of the respiratory distress syndrome in premature infants. Pediatrics, Springfield *50:* 515 (1972).

15 Farrell, P.M.; Kotas, R.V.: The prevention of hyaline membrane disease. New concepts and approaches to therapy. Adv. Pediat. 23: 213 (1976).

16 Fargier, P.; Salle, B.; Baud, M.; et al.: Prévention du syndrome de détresse respiratoire chez le prématuré. Nouv. Presse méd. 3: 1595 (1974).

17 Nathan, D.M.: The respiratory distress syndrome and glucocorticoid treatment. The case for enzyme induction. Mt Sinai J. Med. 42: 150 (1975).

18 Ballard, R.A.; Ballard, P.L.: Use of prenatal glucocorticoid therapy to prevent respiratory distress syndrome. Am. J. Dis. Child. 130: 982 (1976).

19 Ekelund, L.; Arvidson, G.; Ohrlander, S.; et al.: Changes in amniotic fluid phospholipids at treatment with glucocorticoids to prevent respiratory distress syndrome. Acta obstet. gynec. scand. 55: 413 (1976).

20 Collaborative group on antenatal steroid therapy: Effect of antenatal dexamethasone administration on the prevention of respiratory distress syndrome. Am. J. Obstet. Gynec. 141: 276 (1981).

21 Gregory, G.A.; Kitterman, J.A.; Phibbs, R.H.; et al.: Treatment of the idiopathic respiratory-distress syndrome with continuous positive airway pressure. New Engl. J. Med. 284: 1333 (1971).

22 Robertson, B.: Surfactant substitution. Experimental models and clinical applications. Lung 158: 57 (1980).

23 Robertson, B.: Lung surfactant for replacement therapy. Clin. Physiol. 3: 97 (1983).

24 Farrell, P.H.; Avery, M.E.: Hyaline membrane disease. Am. Rev. resp. Dis. 111: 657 (1975).

25 Auld, P.A.M.: Respiratory distress syndromes of the newborn; in Scarpelli, Auld, Goldman, Pulmonary disease of the fetus, newborn and child, p. 447 (Lea & Febiger, Philadelphia 1978).

26 Strang, L.B.: Neonatal respiration, p. 181 (Blackwell, Oxford 1981).

27 Avery, M.E.; Fletcher, B.D.; Williams, R.G.: The lung and its disorders in the newborn infant; 4th ed., p. 222 (Saunders, Philadelphia 1981).

28 Villee, C.A.; Villee, D.B.; Zuckerman, J.: Respiratory distress syndrome (Academic Press, New York 1973).

29 Raivio, K.O.; Hallman, N.; Kouvalainen, K.; Välimäki, I.: Respiratory distress syndrome (Academic Press, London 1984).

30 Farrell, P.M.: Lung development. Biological and clinical perspectives, vol. 2. Neonatal respiratory distress (Academic Press, New York 1982).

31 Hjalmarson, O.: Epidemiology and classification of acute, neonatal respiratory disorders. Acta paediat. scand. 70: 773 (1981).

32 Avery, M.E.: Can RDS be eradicated?, in Raivio, Hallman, Kouvalainen, Välimäki, Respiratory distress syndrome, p. 411 (Academic Press, London 1984).

33 Northway, W.H., Jr.; Rosan, R.C.; Porter, D.Y.: Pulmonary disease following respirator therapy of hyaline membrane disease. Bronchopulmonary dysplasia. New Engl. J. Med. 276: 357 (1967).

34 Robertson, B.: Review of experimental hyaline membrane disease. Diagn. Histopath. 4: 49 (1981).

35 Adams, F.H.; Fujiwara, T.; Latta, H.: 'Alveolar' and whole lung phospholipids of premature newborn lambs. Biol. Neonate 17: 198 (1971).

36 Jobe, A.; Ikegami, M.; Jacobs, H.; et al.: Surfactant pool sizes and severity of RDS in prematurely delivered lambs. Am. Rev. resp. Dis. 127: 751 (1983).

37 Clements, J.A.; Brown, E.S.; Johnson, R.P.: Pulmonary surface tension and the mucus lining of the lungs. Some theoretical considerations. J. appl. Physiol. *12:* 262 (1958).

38 Clements, J.A.; Hustead, R.F.; Johnson, R.P.; et al.: Pulmonary surface tension and alveolar stability. J. appl. Physiol. *16:* 444 (1961).

39 Clements, J.A.: Functions of the alveolar lining. Am. Rev. resp. Dis. *115:* 67 (1977).

40 Guyton, A.C.; Moffat, D.S.: Role of surface tension and surfactant in the transepithelial movement of fluid and in the development of pulmonary edema. Prog. Resp. Res. *15:* 62 (1981).

41 Gruenwald, P.: Surface tension as a factor in the resistance of neonatal lungs to aeration. Am. J. Obstet. Gynec. *53:* 996 (1947).

42 Agostoni, E.; Taglietti, A.; Agostoni, A.; et al.: Mechanical aspects of the first breath. J. appl. Physiol. *13:* 344 (1958).

43 Enhörning, G.; Robertson, B.: Lung expansion in the premature rabbit fetus after tracheal deposition of surfactant. Pediatrics, Springfield *50:* 58 (1972).

44 King, R.J.; Clements, J.A.: Surface active materials from dog lung. III. Thermal analysis. Am. J. Physiol. *223:* 727 (1972).

45 Bangham, A.D.; Morley, C.J.; Phillips, M.C.: The physical properties of an effective lung surfactant. Biochim. biophys. Acta *573:* 552 (1979).

46 Notter, R.H.; Taubold, R.; Davis, R.D.: Hysteresis in saturated phospholipid films and its potential relevance for lung surfactant function in vivo. Expl Lung Res. *3:* 109 (1982).

47 Mead, J.A.; Takishima, T.; Leith, D.: Stress distribution in lungs. A model of pulmonary elasticity. J. appl. Physiol. *28:* 596 (1970).

48 Van Golde, L.M.G.: Metabolism of phospholipids in the lung. Am. Rev. resp. Dis. *114:* 977 (1976).

49 Ohno, K.; Akino, T.; Fujiwara, T.: Phospholipid metabolism in perinatal lung; in Scarpelli, Cosmi, Reviews in perinatal medicine, vol. 2, p. 227 (Raven Press, New York 1978).

50 Batenburg, J.J.; Longmore, W.J.; Van Golde, L.M.G.: The synthesis of phosphatidylcholine by adult rat lung alveolar type II epithelial cells in primary culture. Biochim. biophys. Acta *529:* 160 (1978).

51 Batenburg, J.J.; Longmore, W.J.; Klazinga, W.; et al.: Lysolecithin acyltransferase and lysolecithin:lysolecithin acyltransferase in adult rat lung alveolar type II epithelial cells. Biochim. biophys. Acta *573:* 136 (1979).

52 Batenburg, J.J.; Van Golde, L.M.G.: Formation of pulmonary surfactant in whole lung and in isolated type II alveolar cells; in Scarpelli, Cosmi, Reviews in perinatal medicine, vol. 3, p. 73 (Raven Press, New York 1979).

53 Batenburg, J.J.; Post, M.; Van Golde, L.M.G.: Synthesis of surfactant lipids: studies with type II alveolar cells isolated from adult rat lung. Prog. Resp. Res. *15:* 1 (1981).

54 Chevalier, G.; Collet, A.J.: In vivo incorporation of choline-^{3}H, leucine-^{3}H and galactose-^{3}H in alveolar type II pneumocytes in relation to surfactant synthesis. A quantitative radioautographic study in mouse by electron microscopy. Anat. Rec. *174:* 289 (1972).

55 Rooney, S.A.; Page-Roberts, B.A.; Motoyama, E.K.: Role of lamellar inclusions in surfactant production. Studies on phospholipid composition and biosynthesis in rat and rabbit lung subcellular fractions. J. Lipid Res. *16:* 418 (1975).

56 Engle, M.J.; Sanders, R.L.; Longmore, W.J.: Phospholipid composition and acyl-transferase activity of lamellar bodies isolated from rat lung. Archs Biochem. Biophys. *173:* 586 (1976).

57 Post, M.; Batenburg, J.J.; Schuurmans, E.A.J.M.; et al.: Lamellar bodies isolated from adult human lung tissue. Expl Lung Res. *3:* 17 (1982).

58 Massaro, G.D.; Massaro, D.: Granular pneumocytes. Electron microscopic radioautographic evidence of intracellular protein transport. Am. Rev. resp. Dis. *105:* 927 (1972).

59 Sueishi, K.; Tanaka, K.; Oda, T.: Immunoultrastructural study of surfactant system. Distribution of specific protein of surface active material in rabbit lung. Lab. Invest. *37:* 136 (1977).

60 Williams, C.H.; Thompson, F.E.; Vail, W.J.: The ultrastructure and composition of the lamellar body. Am. Rev. resp. Dis. *111:* 925 (1975).

61 Enhörning, G.; Chamberlain, D.; Contreras, C.; et al.: Isoxsuprine-induced release of pulmonary surfactant in the rabbit fetus. Am. J. Obstet. Gynec. *129:* 197 (1977).

62 Dobbs, L.G.; Mason, R.J.: Pulmonary alveolar type II cells isolated from rats. Release of phosphatidylcholine in response to beta-adrenergic stimulation. J. clin. Invest. *63:* 378 (1979).

63 Novy, M.J.; Portman, O.W.; Bell, M.: Evidence for pulmonary and other sources of amniotic fluid phospholipids in the rhesus monkey; in Villee, Villee, Zuckerman, Respiratory distress syndrome, p. 205 (Academic Press, New York 1973).

64 Grathwohl, C.; Newman, G.E.; Phizackerley, P.J.R.; et al.: Structural studies on lamellated osmiophilic bodies isolated from pig lung. ^{31}P NMR results and water content. Biochim. biophys. Acta *552:* 509 (1979).

65 Morley, C.J.; Bangham, A.D.; Johnson, P.; et al.: Physical and physiological properties of dry lung surfactant. Nature, Lond. *271:* 162 (1978).

66 Weibel, E.R.; Kistler, G.S.; Töndury, G.: A stereologic electron microscopic study of 'tubular myelin figures' in alveolar fluids of rat lungs. Z. Zellforsch. *69:* 418 (1966).

67 Harrison, G.A.; Weibel, J.: The membranous component of alveolar exsudate. J. ultrastruct. Res. *24:* 334 (1968).

68 Gil, J.; Weibel, E.R.: Improvements in demonstration of lining layer of lung alveoli by electron microscopy. Resp. Physiol. *8:* 13 (1969).

69 Stratton, C.J.: The three-dimensional aspect of the mammalian lung surfactant myelin figure. Tissue Cell *9:* 285 (1977).

70 Stratton, C.J.: The periodicity and architecture of lipid retained and extracted lung surfactant and its origin from multilamellar bodies. Tissue Cell *9:* 301 (1977).

71 Williams, M.C.: Conversion of lamellar body membranes into tubular myelin in alveoli of fetal rat lungs. J. Cell Biol. *72:* 260 (1977).

72 Kikkawa, Y.; Manabe, T.: The freeze-fracture study of alveolar type II cells and alveolar content in fetal rabbit lung. Anat. Rec. *190:* 627 (1978).

73 Williams, M.C.: Freeze-fracture studies of tubular myelin and lamellar bodies in fetal and adult rat lungs. J. ultrastruc. Res. *64:* 352 (1978).

74 Sanders, R.L.; Hassett, R.J.; Vatter, A.E.: Isolation of lung lamellar bodies and their conversion to tubular myelin figures in vitro. Anat. Rec. *198:* 485 (1980).

75 Benson, B.J.; Williams, M.C.; Hawgood, S.; et al.: Role of lung surfactant-specific proteins in surfactant structure and function. Prog. Resp. Res. *18:* 83 (1984).

76   Paul, G.W.; Hassett, R.J.; Reiss, O.K.: Formation on lung surfactant films from intact lamellar bodies. Proc. natn. Acad. Sci. USA *74:* 3617 (1977).

77   Hassett, R.J.; Engleman, W.; Kuhn, C.: Extramembranous particles in tubular myelin from rat lung. J. ultrastruct. Res. *71:* 60 (1980).

78   King, R.J.; Macbeth, M.C.: Physicochemical properties of dipalmitoyl phosphatidyl-choline after interaction with an apolipoprotein of pulmonary surfactant. Biochim. biophys. Acta *19:* 86 (1979).

79   Suzuki, Y.: Effect of protein, cholesterol, and phosphatidylglycerol on the surface activity of the lipid-protein complex reconstituted from pig pulmonary surfactant. J. Lipid Res. *23:* 62 (1982).

80   Takahashi, A.; Fujiwara, T.: Proteolipid in bovine lung surfactant: its role in surfactant function. Biochem. biophys. Res. Commun. *135:* 527 (1986).

81   Weibel, E.R.; Gil, J.: Electron microscopic demonstration of an extracellular duplex lining layer of alveoli. Resp. Physiol. *4:* 42 (1968).

82   Kikkawa, Y.: Morphology of alveolar lining layer. Anat. Rec. *167:* 389 (1970).

83   Untersee, P.; Gil, J.; Weibel, E.R.: Visualization of extracellular lining layer of lung alveoli by freeze-etching. Resp. Physiol. *13:* 171 (1971).

84   Roth, J.; Winkelmann, H.; Meyer, H.W.: Electron microscopic studies in mammalian lungs by freeze-etching. IV. Formation of the superficial layer of the surfactant system by lamellar bodies. Exp. Pathol., Suppl. *8:* 354 (1973).

85   Gross, P.; Pfitzer, E.A.; Hatch, T.F.: Alveolar clearance. Its relation to lesions of the respiratory bronchiole. Am. Rev. resp. Dis. *94:* 10 (1966).

86   Kilburn, K.H.: A hypothesis for pulmonary clearance and its implications. Am. Rev. resp. Dis. *98:* 449 (1968).

87   Mendenhall, R.M.: Surface spreading of lung alveolar surfactant. Resp. Physiol. *16:* 175 (1972).

88   Gil, J.; Weibel, E.R.: Extracellular lining of bronchioles after perfusion-fixation of rat lungs for electron microscopy. Anat. Rec. *169:* 185 (1971).

89   Desai, R.; Tetley, T.D.; Curtis, C.G.; et al.: Studies on the fate of pulmonary surfactant in the lung. Biochem. J. *176:* 455 (1978).

90   Zeligs, B.J.; Nerurkar, L.S.; Bellanti, J.A.; et al.: Maturation of rabbit alveolar macrophage during animal development. I. Perinatal influx into alveoli and ultrastructural differentiation. Pediat. Res. *11:* 197 (1977).

91   Nerurkar, L.S.; Zeligs, B.J.; Bellanti, J.A.: Maturation of the rabbit alveolar macrophage during animal development. II. Biochemical and enzymatic changes. Pediat. Res. *11:* 1202 (1977).

92   LaForce, F.M.: Effect of alveolar lining material on phagocytic and bactericidal activity of lung macrophages against *Staphylococcus aureus.* J. lab. clin. Med. *88:* 691 (1976).

93   O'Neill, S.; Lesperance, E.; Klass, D.J.: Rat lung lavage surfactant enhances bacterial phagocytosis and intracellular killing by alveolar macrophages. Am. Rev. resp. Dis. *130:* 225 (1984).

94   Hallman, M.; Epstein, B.L.; Gluck, L.: Analysis of labeling and clearance of lung surfactant phospholipids in rabbit. Evidence of bidirectional surfactant flux between lamellar bodies and alveolar lavage. J. clin. Invest. *68:* 742 (1981).

95   Glatz, T.; Ikegami, M.; Jobe, A.: Metabolism of exogenously administered natural surfactant in the newborn lamb. Pediat. Res. *16:* 711 (1982).

96 Jacobs, H.; Jobe, A.; Ikegami, M.; et al.: The significance of reutilization of surfactant phosphatidylcholine in 3-day-old rabbit. J. biol. Chem. *258:* 4159 (1983).

97 Jacobs, H.; Jobe, A.; Ikegami, M.; et al.: Surfactant phosphatidylcholine source, fluxes, and turnover times in 3-day-old, 10-day-old, and adult rabbits. J. biol. Chem. *4:* 1805 (1982).

98 Albon, N.; Sturtevant, J.M.: Nature of the gel to liquid crystal transition of synthetic phosphatidylcholines. Proc. natn. Acad. Sci. USA *75:* 2258 (1978).

99 Träuble, H.; Eibl, H.; Sawada, H.: Respiration – a critical phenomenon? Lipid phase transitions in the lung alveolar surfactant. Naturwissenschaften *61:* 344 (1974).

100 Ikegami, M.; Jacobs, H.; Jobe, A.: Surfactant function in respiratory distress syndrome. J. Pediat. *102:* 443 (1983).

101 Gruenwald, P.: Normal and abnormal expansion of the lungs of newborn infants obtained at autopsy. I. Expansion of lungs by liquid media. Anat. Rec. *139:* 471 (1961).

102 Gruenwald, P.; Johnson, R.P.; Hustead, R.F.; et al.: Correlation of mechanical properties of infant lungs with surface activity of extracts. Proc. Soc. exp. Biol. Med. *109:* 369 (1962).

103 Gruenwald, P.: Normal and abnormal expansion of the lungs of newborn infants obtained at autopsy. II. Opening pressure, maximal volume, and stability of expansion. Lab. Invest. *12:* 563 (1963).

104 Gruenwald, P.: Normal and abnormal expansion of the lungs of newborn infants obtained at autopsy. III. The pattern of aeration as affected by gestational and postnatal age. Anat. Rec. *146:* 337 (1963).

105 Gruenwald, P.: A numerical index of the stability of lung expansion. J. appl. Physiol. *18:* 665 (1963).

106 Gruenwald, P.; Nitowsky, H.M.; Siegel, I.A.: Respiratory distress syndrome. Perinatal mortality conference. N.Y. State J. Med. *63:* 277 (1963).

107 Enhörning, G.: Photography of peripheral pulmonary airway expansion as affected by surfactant. J. appl. Physiol. *42:* 976 (1977).

108 Grossmann, G.: Expansion pattern of terminal airspaces in the premature rabbit lung after tracheal deposition of surfactant. Pflügers Arch. *367:* 205 (1977).

109 Scarpelli, E.M.; Clutario, B.C.; Traver, D.: Failure of immature lung to produce foam and retain air at birth. Pediat. Res. *13:* 1285 (1979).

110 Scarpelli, E.M.; Kumar, A.; Doyle, C.; et al.: Functional anatomy and volume-pressure characteristics of immature lungs. Resp. Physiol. *45:* 25 (1981).

111 Cook, C.D.; Sutherland, J.M.; Segal, S.; et al.: Studies of respiratory physiology in the newborn infant. III. Measurements of the mechanics of respiration. J. clin. Invest. *36:* 440 (1957).

112 Chu, J.; Clements, J.A.; Cotton, E.; et al.: Neonatal pulmonary ischemia. I. Clinical and physiological study. Pediatrics, Springfield *40:* 709 (1967).

113 Krauss, A.N.; Auld, P.A.M.: Measurement of functional residual capacity in distressed neonates by helium breathing. J. Pediat. *77:* 228 (1970).

114 Tori, C.A.; Krauss, A.N.; Auld, P.A.M.: Serial studies of lung volume and $\dot{V}A/\dot{Q}$ in hyaline membrane disease. Pediat. Res. *7:* 82 (1973).

115 Hjalmarson, O.: Mechanics of breathing in newborn infants with pulmonary disease. Acta paediat. scand., suppl 247 (1974).

116 Hjalmarson, O.: Mechanics of breathing in IRDS; in Raivio, Hallman, Kouvalainen, Välimäki, Respiratory distress syndrome, p. 171 (Academic Press, New York 1984).

117 Nilsson, R.: Lung compliance and lung morphology following artificial ventilation in the premature and full-term rabbit neonate. Scand. J. resp. Dis. *60:* 206 (1979).

118 Nilsson, R.: The artificially ventilated preterm rabbit neonate as experimental model of hyaline membrane disease. Acta anaesth. scand. *26:* 89 (1982).

119 Nilsson, R.; Grossmann, G.; Robertson, B.: Lung surfactant and the pathogenesis of neonatal bronchiolar lesions induced by artificial ventilation. Pediat. Res. *12:* 249 (1978).

120 Harrison, V.C.; Heese, H. de V.; Klein, M.: The significance of grunting in hyaline membrane disease. Pediatrics, Springfield *41:* 549 (1968).

121 Büky, B.; Görgenyi, A.: Idiopathic respiratory distress syndrome. Acoustic, laryngoscopic and radiological investigation. Acta paediat. Acad. Sci. hung. *17:* 219 (1976).

122 Schneeberger, E.E.: Ultrastructural basis for alveolar-capillary permeability to protein; in Porter, O'Connor, Lung liquids. Ciba Fdn Symp. *38:* 3 (1976).

123 Williams, M.C.: Development of the alveolar structure of the fetal rat in late gestation. Fed. Proc. *36:* 2653 (1977).

124 Strang, L.B.: Heterogeneity of pathogenic mechanisms in hyaline membrane disease; in Bloom, Sinclair, Warshaw, The surfactant system and the neonatal lung. Mead Johnson Symposium on Perinatal and Developmental Medicine, No. 14, p. 53 (Mead Johnson & Co, Evansville 1979).

125 Jobe, A.; Ikegami, M.; Jacobs, H.; et al.: Permeability of premature lamb lungs to protein and the effect of surfactant on that permeability. J. appl. Physiol. *55:* 169 (1983).

126 Robertson, B.: Current and counter-current theories on lung surfactant. Scand. J. resp. Dis. *57:* 199 (1976).

127 Tregillus, J.: The asphyxial membrane in the lungs of liveborn infants. J. Obstet. Gynaec. Br. Emp. *58:* 406 (1951).

128 Barter, R.A.: The neonatal pulmonary hyaline membrane. Lancet *ii:* 160 (1959).

129 Barter, R.A.; Maddison, T.G.: The nature of the neonatal pulmonary hyaline membrane. Archs Dis. Childh. *35:* 460 (1960).

130 Taghizadeh, A.; Reynolds, E.O.R.: Pathogenesis of bronchopulmonary dysplasia following hyaline membrane disease. Am. J. Path. *82:* 241 (1976).

131 Robertson, B.: Lung morphology in clinical and experimental RDS: effect of treatment with supplementary surfactant. Wiss. Z. Humboldt-Universität Berlin Math-Nat. R. *29:* 597 (1980).

132 Finlay-Jones, J.M.; Papadimitriou, J.M.; Barter, R.A.: Pulmonary hyaline membrane. Light and electron microscopic study of the early stage. J. Path. *112:* 117 (1974).

133 Van Breemen, V.L.; Neustein, H.B.; Bruns, P.D.: Pulmonary hyaline membranes studied with the electron microscope. Am. J. Path. *33:* 769 (1957).

134 Campiche, M.; Prod'hom, S.; Gauthier, A.: Etude au microscope électronique du poumon de prématurés morts en détresse respiratoire. Annls paediat. *196:* 81 (1961).

135 Campiche, M.; Jacotet, M.; Juillard, E.: La pneumatose à membranes hyalines. Observations au microscope électronique. Annls paediat. *199:* 74 (1962).

136 Gandy, G.; Jacobson, W.; Gairdner, D.: Hyaline membrane disease. I. Cellular changes. Archs Dis. Childh. *45:* 289 (1970).

137 Lauweryns, J.: 'Hyaline membrane disease' in newborn infants. Macroscopic, radiographic, and light and electron microscopic studies. Human Pathol. *1:* 175 (1970).

138 Cutz, E.; Chan, W.: Correlative light (LM), transmission (TEM) and scanning electron microscopic (SEM) study of hyaline membrane disease (HMD). Scanning electron

microscopy, 1976, part V. Proc. Workshop on Advances in Biomedical Application of the SEM, IIT Research Institute, Chicago 1976, p. 239.

139   Manabe, T.: Ultrastructural observation of neonatal lungs with transmission electron microscope and freeze-fracture replication. Acta path. jap. *31:* 979 (1981).

140   Gruenwald, P.: The significance of pulmonary hyaline membranes in newborn infants. J. Am. med. Ass. *166:* 621 (1958).

141   Angerwall, L.; Edström, J.E.: The occurrence of deoxyribonucleic acid in pulmonary hyaline membranes of the newborn infant. Acta pathol. microbiol. scand. *44:* 1 (1958).

142   Gitlin, D.; Craig, J.M.: The nature of the hyaline membrane in asphyxia of the newborn. Pediatrics, Springfield *17:* 64 (1956).

143   Cho, S.Y.; Sastre, M.: Pulmonary yellow hyaline membrane disease. New variant in premature infants with intrahepatic cholestasis. Archs Pathol. Lab. Med. *100:* 145 (1976).

144   Robertson, B.: Pulmonary hyaline membranes of the newborn. The structure of the membranes at varying postnatal age. Acta pathol. microbiol. scand. *62:* 581 (1964).

145   Craig, J.M.; Fenton, K.; Gitlin, D.: Obstructive factors in the pulmonary hyaline membrane syndrome in asphyxia of the newborn. Pediatrics, Springfield *22:* 847 (1958).

146   Lachmann, B.; Tischer, A.M.; Grossmann, G.; et al.: Lung compliance and alveolar expansion in the artificially ventilated premature newborn rabbit after maternal treatment with ambroxol. Respiration *42:* 209 (1981).

147   Chu, J.; Clements, J.A.; Cotton, E.; et al.: The pulmonary hypoperfusion syndrome. Pediatrics, Springfield *35:* 733 (1965).

148   Krahl, V.E.: Evidence of pulmonary arteriolar constriction and arteriovenous shunting in pulmonary hypoperfusion syndrome (respiratory distress syndrome of the newborn). Adv. Microcirc. *2:* 1 (1969).

149   Swyer, P.R.; Murdock, A.I.; Llewellyn, M.A.; et al.: Right to left shunting in the respiratory distress syndrome of the newborn. Bull. Physiopathol. Resp. *9:* 1495 (1973).

150   Strang, L.B.; McLeish, M.H.: Ventilatory failure and right to left shunts in newborn infants with respiratory distress. Pediatrics, Springfield *28:* 17 (1961).

151   Roberton, N.R.C.; Dahlenburg, G.W.: Ductus arteriosus shunts in the respiratory distress syndrome. Pediat. Res. *3:* 149 (1969).

152   Lauweryns, J.; Bonte, J.; Van der Schueren, G.: A haemodynamic study of the syndrome of secondary pulmonary atelectasis. Acta anat. *46:* 142 (1961).

153   Lauweryns, J.M.: Pulmonary arterial vasculature in neonatal hyaline membrane disease. Science *153:* 1275 (1966).

154   Ivemark, B.; Wallgren, G.: The pulmonary vascular pattern in idiopathic respiratory distress. A micro-angiographic study. Acta pathol. microbiol. scand. *76:* 203 (1969).

155   Oeberius Kapteyn, J.L.T.; Wolvius, G.G.; Wagenvoort, C.A.: The pulmonary arteries and arterioles in hyaline membrane disease. Archs Dis. Childh. *38:* 468 (1963).

156   Naeye, R.L.: Pulmonary arterial abnormalities associated with hyaline membrane disease. Am. J. Path. *48:* 869 (1966).

157   Lauweryns, J.M.: Hyaline membrane disease: a pathological study of 55 infants. Archs Dis. Childh. *40:* 618 (1965).

158   Lauweryns, J.M.; Claessens, St.; Boussauw, L.: The pulmonary lymphatics in neonatal hyaline membrane disease. Pediatrics, Springfield *41:* 917 (1968).

159   Humphreys, P.W.; Normand, I.C.S.; Reynolds, E.O.R.; et al.: Pulmonary lymph flow and the uptake of liquid from the lungs of the lamb at the start of breathing. J. Physiol. *193:* 1 (1967).

160 Normand, I.C.S.; Reynolds, E.O.R.; Strang, L.B.; et al.: Flow and protein concentration of lymph flow from the lungs of lambs developing hyaline membrane disease. Archs Dis. Childh. *43:* 334 (1968).

161 Boss, J.H.; Craig, J.M.: Reparative phenomena in lungs of neonates with hyaline membranes. Pediatrics, Springfield *29:* 890 (1962).

162 Robertson, B.; Tunell, R.; Rudhe, U.: Late stages of pulmonary hyaline membranes of the newborn. Acta paediat. scand. *53:* 433 (1964).

163 Barter, R.A.; Byrne, M.J.; Carter, R.F.: Pulmonary hyaline membranes. Late results of injury to lung linings. Archs Dis. Childh. *41:* 489 (1966).

164 Becker, M.J.; Koppe, J.G.: Pulmonary structural changes in neonatal hyaline membrane disease treated with high pressure artificial respiration. Thorax *24:* 689 (1969).

165 Larroche, J.C.; Nessmann, C.; Bennoun, M.: La maladie des membranes hyalines: évolution, cicatrisation, séquelles. Etude histologique. Archs fr. pediat. *28:* 113 (1971).

166 Northway, W.H., Jr.; Rosan, R.C.: Radiographic features of pulmonary oxygen toxicity in the newborn; bronchopulmonary dysplasia. Radiology *91:* 49 (1968).

167 Shepard, F.M.; Johnston, R.B., Jr.; Klatte, E.C.; et al.: Residual pulmonary findings in clinical hyaline membrane disease. New Engl. J. Med. *279:* 1063 (1968).

168 Pusey, V.A.; MacPherson, R.I.; Chernick, V.: Pulmonary fibroplasia following prolonged artificial ventilation of newborn infants. Can. med. Ass. J. *100:* 451 (1969).

169 Anderson, W.R.; Strickland, M.B.: Pulmonary complications of oxygen therapy in the neonate. Post-mortem study of bronchopulmonary dysplasia with emphasis on fibroproliferative bronchitis and bronchiolitis. Archs Path. *91:* 506 (1971).

170 Banerjee, C.K.; Girling, D.J.; Wigglesworth, J.S.: Pulmonary fibroplasia in newborn babies treated with oxygen and artificial ventilation. Archs Dis. Childh. *47:* 509 (1972).

171 Anderson, W.R.; Strickland, M.B.; Tsai, S.H.; et al.: Light microscopic and ultrastructural study of the adverse effects of oxygen therapy on the neonate lung. Am. J. Path. *73:* 327 (1973).

172 Bomsel, F.; Couchard, M.; Polje, J.; et al.: Pulmonary sequelae of the hyaline membrane disease. Iatrogenic factors? Radiological and anatomical study. Ann. Radiol. *16:* 70 (1973).

173 Rosan, R.C.: Hyaline membrane disease and a related spectrum of neonatal pneumopathies. Perspect. pediatr. Pathol. *2:* 15 (1975).

174 Bonikos, D.S.; Bensch, K.G.; Northway, W.H., Jr.; et al.: Bronchopulmonary dysplasia: the pulmonary pathologic sequel of necrotizing bronchiolitis and pulmonary fibrosis. Human Pathol. *7:* 643 (1976).

175 Gautier, A.; Campiche, M.; Bozic, C.; et al.: Pulmonary epithelium in the human fetus and newborn. 5th Int. Congr. Electron Microscopy, vol. 2 (Academic Press, New York 1962).

176 Balis, J.U.; Delivora, M.; Conen, P.E.: Maturation of postnatal human lung and the idiopathic respiratory distress syndrome. Lab. Invest. *15:* 530 (1966).

177 Lindroth, M.; Svenningsen, N.W.; Ahlström, H.; et al.: Evaluation of mechanical ventilation in newborn infants. II. Pulmonary and neuro-developmental sequelae in relation to original diagnosis. Acta paediat. scand. *69:* 151 (1980).

178 Weissner, K.; Ganz, R.; Olafsson, A.; et al.: Bronchopulmonary dysplasia in the premature baby. Respiration *27:* 36 (1970).

179 Sobonya, R.E.; Logvinoff, M.M.; Taussig, L.M.; et al.: Morphometric analysis of the lung in prolonged bronchopulmonary dysplasia. Pediat. Res. *16:* 969 (1982).

180 Johnson, D.E.; Lock, J.E.; Elde, R.P.; et al.: Pulmonary neuroendocrine cells in hyaline membrane disease and bronchopulmonary dysplasia. Pediat. Res. *16:* 446 (1982).
181 Ahlström, H.; Mortensson, W.; Robertson, B.: Reversibility of bronchiolar and alveolar lesions in bronchopulmonary dysplasia. Opuscula Med. *29:* 102 (1984).
182 Stocks, J.; Godfrey, S.: The role of artificial ventilation, oxygen and CPAP in the pathogenesis of lung damage in neonates. Pediatrics, Springfield *57:* 352 (1976).
183 Stocks, J.; Godfrey, S.; Reynolds, E.O.R.: Airway resistance in infants after various treatments for hyaline membrane disease. Special emphasis on prolonged high levels of inspired oxygen. Pediatrics, Springfield *61:* 178 (1978).
184 Stahlman, M.: Long time results of respirator therapy. Biol. Neonate *16:* 133 (1970).
185 Philip, A.G.S.: Oxygen plus pressure plus time: the etiology of bronchopulmonary dysplasia. Pediatrics, Springfield *55:* 44 (1975).
186 Wilson, M.G.; Mikity, V.G.: A new form of respiratory disease in premature infants. Am. J. Dis. Child. *99:* 489 (1960).
187 Baghdassarian, O.M.; Avery, M.E.; Neuhauser, E.B.D.: A form of pulmonary insufficiency in premature infants; pulmonary dysmaturity? Am. J. Roentgenol. *89:* 1020 (1963).
188 Swyer, P.R.; Delivora-Papadopoulos, M.; Levison, H.; et al.: The pulmonary syndrome of Wilson and Mikity. Pediatrics, Springfield *36:* 374 (1965).
189 Hodgman, J.E.; Mikity, G.; Tatter, D.; et al.: Chronic respiratory distress in the premature infant. Wilson-Mikity syndrome. Pediatrics, Springfield *44:* 179 (1969).
190 Avery, M.E.; Fletcher, B.D.; Williams, R.G.: The lung and its disorders in the newborn infant; 4th ed., p. 263 (Saunders, Philadelphia 1981).
191 Merritt, T.A.; Puccia, J.M.; Stuard, I.D.: Cytologic evaluation of pulmonary effluent in neonates with respiratory distress syndrome and bronchopulmonary dysplasia. Acta cytol. *6:* 631 (1981).
192 Merritt, T.A.; Stuard, I.D.; Puccia, J.; et al.: Newborn tracheal aspirate cytology: classification during respiratory distress syndrome and bronchopulmonary dysplasia. J. Pediat. *98:* 949 (1981).
193 Doshi, N.; Kanbour, A.; Fujikura, T.; et al.: Tracheal aspiration cytology in neonates with respiratory distress. Histopathologic correlation. Acta cytol. *26:* 15 (1982).
194 Gluck, L.; Motoyama, E.K.; Smith, H.L.; et al.: The biochemical development of surface activity in mammalian lung. I. The surface active phospholipids; the separation and distribution of surface active lecithin in the lung of the developing rabbit fetus. Pediat. Res. *1:* 237 (1967).
195 Gluck, L.; Sribney, M.; Kulovich, M.V.: The biochemical development of surface activity in mammalian lung. II. The biosynthesis of phospholipids in the lung of the developing rabbit fetus and newborn. Pediat. Res. *1:* 247 (1967).
196 Kikkawa, Y.; Motoyama, E.K.; Gluck, L.: Study of lungs of fetal and newborn rabbits. Morphologic, biochemical and surface physical development. Am. J. Path. *52:* 177 (1968).
197 Gluck, L.; Landowne, R.A.; Kulovich, M.V.: Biochemical development of surface activity in mammalian lung. III. Structural changes in lung lecithin during development of the rabbit fetus and newborn. Pediat. Res. *4:* 352 (1970).
198 Miller, H.C.; Futrakul, P.: Birth weight, gestational age, and sex as determining factors in the incidence of respiratory distress syndrome of prematurely born infants. J. Pediat. *72:* 628 (1968).

199 Naeye, R.L.; Burt, L.S.; Wright, D.L.; et al.: Neonatal mortality. The male disadvantage. Pediatrics, Springfield *48:* 902 (1971).

200 Naeye, R.L.; Freeman, R.K.; Blanc, W.A.: Nutrition, sex, and fetal lung maturation. Pediat. Res. *8:* 200 (1974).

201 Torday, J.S.; Nielsen, H.C.; Fencl, M. de M.; et al.: Sex differences in fetal lung maturation. Am. Rev. resp. Dis. *123:* 205 (1981).

202 Kotas, R.V.; Avery, M.E.: The influence of sex on fetal rabbit lung maturation and on the response to glucocorticoid. Am. Rev. resp. Dis. *121:* 377 (1980).

203 Nielsen, H.C.; Torday, J.S.: Sex differences in fetal rabbit pulmonary surfactant production. Pediat. Res. *15:* 1245 (1981).

204 Lachmann, B.; Grossmann, G.; Nilsson, R.; et al.: Lung mechanics during spontaneous ventilation in premature and fullterm rabbit neonates. Resp. Physiol. *38:* 283 (1979).

205 Nilsson, R.; Grossmann, G.; Robertson, B.: Bronchiolar epithelial lesions induced in the premature rabbit neonate by short periods of artificial ventilation. Acta pathol. microbiol. scand., A, Pathol. *88:* 359 (1980).

206 Nilsson, R.; Robertson, B.: Bronchiolar epithelial lesions in spontaneously breathing premature newborn rabbits. Biol. Neonate *48:* 357 (1985).

207 Humphreys, P.W.; Strang, L.B.: Effects of gestation and prenatal asphyxia on pulmonary surface properties of the foetal rabbit. J. Physiol. Lond. *192:* 53 (1967).

208 Nilsson, R.; Grossmann, G.; Robertson, B.: Pathogenesis of neonatal lung lesions induced by artificial ventilation; evidence against the role of barotrauma. Respiration *40:* 218 (1980).

209 Enhörning, G.; Grossmann, G.; Robertson, B.: Tracheal deposition of surfactant before the first breath. Am. Rev. resp. Dis. *107:* 921 (1973).

210 Robertson, B.; Enhörning, G.: The alveolar lining of the premature newborn rabbit after pharyngeal deposition of surfactant. Lab. Invest. *31:* 54 (1974).

211 Robertson, B.; Berry, D.; Curstedt, T.; et al.: Leakage of protein in the immature rabbit lung; the effect of surfactant replacement. Resp. Physiol. *61:* 265 (1985).

212 Nilsson, R.; Grossmann, G.; Berggren, P.; et al.: Surfactant treatment in experimental hyaline membrane disease. Eur. J. resp. Dis. *62:* 441 (1981).

213 Lachmann, B.; Grossmann, G.; Freyse, J.; et al.: Lung-thorax compliance in the artificially ventilated premature rabbit neonate in relation to variations in inspiration: expiration ratio. Pediat. Res. *15:* 833 (1981).

214 Reynolds, E.O.R.: Effect of alterations in mechanical ventilator setting on pulmonary gas exchange in hyaline membrane disease. Archs Dis. Childh. *46:* 152 (1971).

215 Herman, S.; Reynolds, E.O.R.: Methods for improving oxygenation in infants ventilated for severe hyaline membrane disease. Archs Dis. Childh. *48:* 612 (1973).

216 Reynolds, E.O.R.; Taghizadeh, A.: Improved prognosis of infants mechanically ventilated for hyaline membrane disease. Archs Dis. Childh. *49:* 505 (1974).

217 Chernick, V.: Mechanics of the first inspiration. Semin. Perinat. *1:* 347 (1977).

218 Avery, M.E.; Fletcher, B.D.; Williams, R.G.: The lung and its disorders in the newborn infant; 4th ed., p. 29 (Saunders, Philadelphia 1981).

219 Lachmann, B.; Berggren, P.; Curstedt, T.; et al.: Combined effects of surfactant substitution and prolongation of inspiration phase in artificially ventilated premature newborn rabbits. Pediat. Res. *16:* 921 (1982).

220 Rigaut, J.P.; Berggren, P.; Robertson, B.: Automated techniques for the study of

lung alveolar stereological parameters with the IBAS image analyser on optical micro-scopy sections. J. Microsc. *130:* 53 (1983).

221 Avery, M.E.: Pharmacological approaches to the acceleration of fetal lung maturation. Br. med. Bull. *31:* 13 (1975).

222 Robertson, B.: Neonatal pulmonary mechanics and morphology after experimental therapeutic regimens; in Scarpelli, Cosmi, Reviews in perinatal medicine, vol. 4, p. 337 (Raven Press, New York 1981).

223 Robertson, B.: Treatment of the premature rabbit neonate with supplementary surfac-tant. Prog. Resp. Res. *15:* 269 (1981).

224 Fujiwara, T.; Maeta, H.; Chida, S.; et al.: Improved pulmonary pressure-volume char-acteristics in premature newborn rabbits after tracheal instillation of artificial surfac-tant. IRCS med. Sci. *7:* 312 (1979).

225 Fujiwara, T.; Maeta, H.; Chida, S.; et al.: Improved lung-thorax compliance and pre-vention of neonatal pulmonary lesion in prematurely delivered rabbit neonates sub-jected to IPPV after tracheal instillation of artificial surfactant. IRCS med. Sci. *7:* 313 (1979).

226 Tanaka, Y.; Takei, T.; Masuda, K.: Lung surfactants. III. Correlations among ac-tivities in vitro, in situ and in vivo, and chemical composition. Chem. pharm. Bull., Tokyo *31:* 4110 (1983).

227 Grossmann, G.; Larsson, I.; Nilsson, R.; et al.: Lung expansion in premature newborn rabbits treated with emulsified synthetic surfactant; principles for experimental evalu-ation of synthetic substitutes for pulmonary surfactant. Respiration *45:* 327 (1984).

228 Morley, C.J.; Robertson, B.; Lachmann, B.; et al.: Artificial surfactant and natural surfactant. Comparative study of the effects on premature rabbit lungs. Archs Dis. Childh. *55:* 758 (1980).

229 Berggren, P.; Curstedt, T.; Grossmann, G.; et al.: Physiological activity of pulmonary surfactant with low protein content; effects of enrichment with synthetic phospholipids. Exp. Lung Res. *8:* 29 (1985).

230 Schneider, H.A.; Hallman, M.; Benirschke, K.; et al.: Human surfactant. A therapeu-tic trial in premature rabbits. J. Pediat. *100:* 619 (1982).

231 Fujiwara, T.; Maeta, H.; Chida, S.; et al.: Artificial surfactant therapy in hyaline-mem-brane disease. Lancet *i:* 55 (1980).

232 Hallman, M.; Merritt, T.A.; Schneider, H.; et al.: Isolation of human surfactant from amniotic fluid and a pilot study of its efficacy in respiratory distress syndrome. Pediat-rics *71:* 473 (1983).

233 Morley, C.; Greenough, A.; Miller, N.; et al.: Cambridge artificial surfactant trial. Prog. Resp. Res. *18:* 274 (1984).

234 Hallman, M.; Merritt, T.A.; Jarvenpaa, A.L.; et al.: Exogenous human surfactant for treatment of severe respiratory distress syndrome: A randomized prospective clinical trial. J. Pediat. *106:* 963 (1985).

235 Adams, F.H.; Towers, B.; Osher, A.B.; et al.: Effects of tracheal instillation of natural surfactant in premature lambs. I. Clinical and autopsy findings. Pediat. Res. *12:* 841 (1978).

236 Ikegami, M.; Adams, F.H.; Towers, B.; et al.: The quantity of natural surfactant necessary to prevent the respiratory distress syndrome in premature lambs. Pediat. Res. *14:* 1082 (1980).

237 Jobe, A.; Ikegami, M.; Glatz, T.; et al.: Duration and characteristics of treatment of premature lambs with natural surfactant. J. clin. Invest. *67:* 370 (1981).

238 Ikegami, M.; Jobe, A.; Jacobs, H.; et al.: Sequential treatment of premature lambs with an artificial surfactant and natural surfactant. J. clin. Invest. *68:* 491 (1981).

239 Jacobs, H.; Jobe, A.; Ikegami, M.; et al.: Premature lambs rescued from respiratory failure with natural surfactant: clinical and biophysical correlates. Pediat. Res. *16:* 424 (1982).

240 Egan, E.A.; Notter, R.H.; Kwong, M.S.; et al.: Natural and artificial lung surfactant replacement therapy in premature lambs. J. appl. Physiol. *55:* 875 (1983).

241 Jobe, A.; Jacobs, H.; Ikegami, M.; et al.: Lung protein leaks in ventilated lambs: effect of gestational age. J. appl. Physiol. *58:* 1246 (1985).

242 Ikegami, M.; Jobe, A.; Glatz, T.: Surface activity following natural surfactant treatment in premature lambs. J. appl. Physiol. *51:* 306 (1981).

243 Ikegami, M.; Jobe, A.; Jacobs, H.; et al.: A protein from airways of premature lambs that inhibits surfactant function. J. appl. Physiol. *57:* 1134 (1984).

244 Ikegami, M.; Jobe, A.; Berry, D.: A protein that inhibits surfactant in respiratory distress syndrome. Biol. Neonate (in press).

245 Enhörning, G.; Hill, D.; Sherwood, G.; et al.: Improved ventilation of prematurely-delivered primates following tracheal deposition of surfactant. Am. J. Obstet. Gynec. *132:* 529 (1978).

246 Cutz, E.; Enhörning, G.; Robertson, B.; et al.: Hyaline membrane disease. Effect of surfactant prophylaxis on lung morphology in premature primates. Am. J. Path. *92:* 581 (1978).

247 Jacobs, R.F.; Wilson, C.B.; Palmer, S.; et al.: Factors related to the appearance of alveolar macrophages in the developing lung. Am. Rev. resp. Dis. *131:* 548 (1985).

248 Bellanti, J.A.; Nerurkar, I.S.; Zelings, B.J.: Host defenses in the fetus and neonate. Studies of the alveolar macrophages during maturation. Pediatrics, Springfield *64:* 726 (1979).

249 Jacob, J.; Edwards, D.; Gluck, L.: Early-onset sepsis and pneumonia observed as respiratory distress syndrome. Am. J. Dis. Child. *134:* 766 (1980).

250 Notter, R.H.; Shapiro, D.L.: Lung surfactant in an era of replacement therapy. Pediatrics, Springfield *68:* 781 (1981).

251 Fujiwara, T.: Surfactant replacement in neonatal RDS; in Robertson, Van Golde, Batenburg, Pulmonary surfactant, p. 479, (Elsevier, Amsterdam 1984).

252 Smyth, J.A.; Metcalfe, I.L.; Duffty, P.; et al.: Hyaline membrane disease treated with bovine surfactant. Pediatrics, Springfield *71:* 913 (1983).

253 Nohara, K.; Muramatsu, K.; Oda, T.: Six cases of RDS treated with Surfactant CK. J. Jap. med. Soc. Biol. Interface *14:* 173 (1983).

254 Robertson, B.; Noack, G.; Bevilacqua, G.; et al.: Surfactant replacement in severe neonatal respiratory distress syndrome; in Vignali, Cosmi, Luerti, Diagnosis and treatment of fetal lung immaturity, p. 193 (Masson, Milano 1986).

Dr. Bengt Robertson, Barnpatologiska Laboratoriet, St. Gorans Sjukhus, Box 12500, S–112 81 Stockholm (Sweden)

Perspect. pediatr. Pathol., vol. 11, pp. 47–81 (Karger, Basel 1987)

Idiopathic Pulmonary Hemosiderosis and Related Disorders in Infancy and Childhood

Ernest Cutz

Department of Pathology, The Hospital for Sick Children and
University of Toronto, Toronto, Ont., Canada

Introduction

Hemosiderin in the lung is a nonspecific finding that usually indicates previous hemorrhage or aspiration of blood. Hemosiderin-laden macrophages can be found in diseases such as inflammation or neoplasia, infection, blood dyscrasia, chronic heart failure, and pulmonary hypertension. Unless massive hemorrhage occurs, the extent of bleeding and subsequent deposition of hemosiderin is limited and rarely a cause of significant clinical symptoms.

More challenging to the clinicians and pathologists is a group of rare disorders in the distal parts of the lung characterized by single or repeated episodes of bleeding that can lead to massive, occasionally fatal, hemorrhage or progress to chronic pulmonary disease. The clinical presentation usually includes hemoptysis, dyspnea, iron deficiency anemia, and transient pulmonary infiltrates. Diffuse pulmonary hemorrhage has been divided into two broad categories on the basis of clinical, laboratory, and immunopathological findings: (a) primary idiopathic pulmonary hemosiderosis (IPH), in which pulmonary hemorrhage is an isolated phenomenon without demonstrable immunologic abnormality or other apparent cause, and (b) secondary pulmonary hemorrhage associated with immunologically mediated renal or vascular disease [1].

Pulmonary hemosiderosis and related disorders in infancy and childhood are reviewed here with main emphasis on histopathology, ultrastructure, immunopathologic findings, and pathogenesis.

Classification

The main reason for classifying pulmonary hemosiderosis is to differentiate IPH from other conditions with better defined or known causes. The diagnosis of IPH is established by exclusion after all known causes of pulmonary hemorrhage have been ruled out. A simple classification of pulmonary hemosiderosis in infancy and childhood includes two main categories: (a) primary (intrinsic to the lung); (b) secondary (related to cardiac or systemic disease) [2]. Morgan and Turner-Warwick [3] listed nine variants of pulmonary hemosiderosis in children and adults, but they cautioned against regarding the variants of pulmonary hemosiderosis as distinct clinicopathological entities since the precise etiology and pathogenesis of many of these conditions have not been defined.

Our classification of pulmonary hemosiderosis in infancy and childhood is based on the differential diagnosis, and it directs a search for underlying disease and etiologic factors (table I).

Idiopathic Pulmonary Hemosiderosis (IPH)

IPH is the commonest amongst the disorders characterized by diffuse pulmonary hemorrhage and hemosiderosis. Although the first description of IPH is credited to Virchow [4], the clinical and pathological features were so clearly defined by Ceelen [5] in 1931, that IPH is sometimes referred to as Ceelen's disease. More than 100 cases have been reported by 1962 [6], and at least as many cases have been recorded since then.

Clinical and Laboratory Findings

Patients with IPH usually present during the first decade of life, but cases presenting during infancy have also been described [7]. In a series reported by Soergel and Sommers, [6], most patients were between the ages of one and seven years, and most adults were less than 30 years old; the oldest patient was 48 years old. Although most cases of IPH are sporadic, some have been familial [8, 9].

The presenting symptoms and outcome of the disease are variable. There is usually no preceding illness, and the family history is often negative. Occult pulmonary bleeding may manifest as chronic, nonproductive cough, dyspnea and iron-deficiency anemia. Cytologic examination of the sputum or a gastric aspirate may reveal hemosiderin-laden macrophages,

Table I. Disorders associated with diffuse pulmonary hemorrhage and hemosiderosis in infancy and childhood

1 Idiopathic pulmonary hemosiderosis (isolated)
2 Pulmonary hemosiderosis associated with sensitivity to cow's milk
3 Pulmonary hemosiderosis and glomerulonephritis
  a With antibodies to GBM (Goodpasture's syndrome)
  b Without antibodies to GBM (usually immune-complex glomerulonephritis)
4 Pulmonary hemosiderosis associated with collagen vascular or purpuric disease
  a Systemic lupus erythematosus
  b Wegener's granulomatosis
  c Polyarteritis nodosa
  d Rheumatoid arthritis
  e Schönlein-Henoch purpura
  f Idiopathic thrombocytopenic purpura
5 Pulmonary hemosiderosis secondary to cardiac disease, intrapulmonary vascular lesions or malformations
  a Chronic left- or right-sided heart failure (i.e. mitral stenosis)
  b Pulmonary hypertension
  c Pulmonary veno occlusive disease
  d Pulmonary lymphangioleiomatosis
  e Arteriovenous fistulas and other congenital vascular malformations
  f Vascular thrombosis with infarction

Modified from Heiner [2] and Morgan and Turner-Warwick [3]. The disorders are listed in the order as they are discussed in the text.

and the stool may contain occult blood derived from swallowed sputum. Some episodes of hemoptysis are fatal [6]. Other clinical symptoms are less specific and include fever, lymphadenopathy, hepatomegaly and splenomegaly.

The radiographic changes depend on the stage of disease [2, 3]. The chest radiograph during an episode of acute hemorrhage is characterized by patchy or diffuse pulmonary infiltrates or occasionally massive confluent shadows that may clear rapidly. Following repeated episodes of pulmonary hemorrhage, there is usually perihilar reticulation or a pattern of diffuse interstitial disease. Nuclear scan imaging of radiolabeled red cells [10] and a test based on carbon-15-labeled carbon monoxide clearance [11] are two recent techniques for studying intrapulmonary hemorrhage.

Laboratory studies commonly reveal an iron-deficiency, microcytic, hypochromic anemia [2, 3, 6], sometimes with extremely low hemoglobin concentration. The bone marrow examination shows reactive erythroid hyperplasia and depleted iron stores. Increased reticulocytes, positive Coombs' test and jaundice in some patients with IPH suggest an element of hemolysis, probably secondary to massive hemorrhage and without a significant pathogenetic role [12].

The levels of serum iron are typically low and the total-iron binding capacity increased. Detailed hematologic and iron kinetic studies exclude abnormalities of the red cells, significant hemolysis, and defects in iron metabolism, indicating that anemia is secondary to blood loss [12]. In some cases, however, the severity of anemia appears greater than would be expected from a relatively small loss of blood into the lung and the discrepancy remains unexplained. The results of pulmonary function tests are variable; some patients have normal function whereas others have impaired diffusion, decreased compliance, and airway obstruction [13]. Serial measurements of pulmonary function are recommended for assessment of disease activity.

In most cases, the diagnosis of IPH can be made on the basis of typical clinical, radiographic and laboratory findings. However, confirmation requires a lung biopsy and a kidney biopsy (if renal function is abnormal) to exclude other disorders associated with pulmonary hemorrhage, particularly renal and collagen-vascular diseases (table I). Most patients with IPH have normal renal function without circulating autoantibodies (e.g. glomerular antibasement membrane antibody, LE cells, antinuclear factor) [12, 14, 15].

The prognosis is uncertain. The cases reported by Soergel and Sommers [6] had a median survival of 3 years. At one extreme are patients who die of massive pulmonary hemorrhage shortly after presentation, at the other, patients who remain in remission for several years. Repeated exacerbations usually lead to chronic pulmonary disease with interstitial fibrosis, pulmonary hypertension, and right-sided heart failure [6].

Seven patients with IPH were seen at our institution during the past 23 years (table II). The overall clinical, radiographic and laboratory findings were similar to those reported by others [6, 12, 14, 15]. The mean age at presentation was 4 years (all patients were less than 10 years of age and none was younger than 2 years). Five patients presented with pulmonary symptoms and moderate to severe iron deficiency anemia, whereas two patients had chronic anemia as the main problem. One patient (case 1, table II) died of massive hemoptysis, 3 years following the first symptoms. Six patients are still alive; 2 have had multiple exacerbations, and the other 4 appear to be symptom-free 3–10 years after presentation. No pa-

Table II. Clinical features of patients with IPH (The Hospital for Sick Children, Toronto 1960–1984)

Case No.	Age at onset years	Sex	Presenting symptoms	Follow-up and current status
1†	6	F	'recurrent pneumonitis' anemia, hemoptysis	death at 9 years due to hemoptysis
2	3.5	F	anemia	relapse at 6½ years; currently 10 years, stable
3	3	F	cough, dyspnea, fever anemia (↑ liver, spleen, LN)	9 years, multiple exacerbations
4	3	M	anemia, fever, jaundice, (↑ cervic. LN)	13 years, stable
5	4	F	cough, fever, anemia	14 years, stable
6	3	M	anemia, cough, dyspnea, hemoptysis	11 years, recurrent attacks
7	5	F	anemia, 'recurrent pneumonia', hemoptysis	8 years, stable
Mean age 4 years		5 F/2 M		mean follow-up 6 years

†=Died; F=female; M=male; LN=lymph nodes.

Table III. Histopathologic findings in lung biopsies of patients with IPH

Case No.	Age at biopsy years	Recent hemorrhage	Hemosiderin deposition			Interstitial fibrosis
			alveolar macrophages	interstitium	elastica	
1	8	3+D	3+D	2+F	2+F	3+D
2*	6.5	3+F	3+D	1+F	–	1–2+F
3	3	1+F	2–3+F	1–2+F	1+F	2–3+F
4	6.5	1–2+F	1–2+F	1+F	–	1+F
5*	4	1–2+F	2–3+F	2–3+F	2–3+F	2–3+F
6*	8	1–2+F	1–2+F	1+F	–	1+F
7*	8	2+F	2+F	1+F	–	1+F

* Cases examined by immunofluorescence and electron microscopy.
F=Focal; D=diffuse; –=absent; 1+=mild; 2+=moderate; 3+=severe.

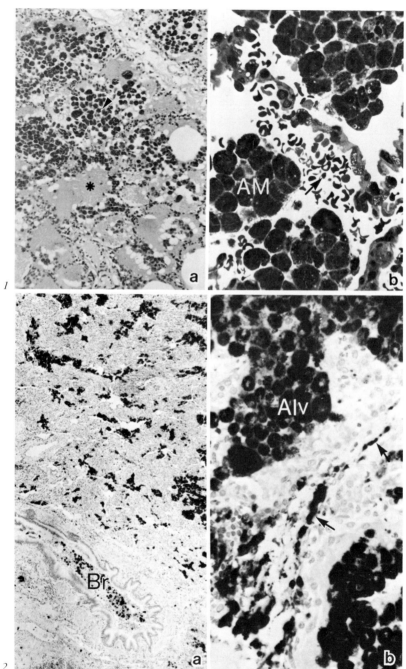

tient had evidence of cardiac, renal or collagen-vascular disease, and none had detectable autoantibodies or positive tests for cow's milk allergy.

Open lung biopsies were performed in all patients, either at the time of presentation or following a subsequent episode of pulmonary bleeding. The samples for light microscopy were fixed in 10% neutral buffered formalin or in Zenker's solution. The sections were stained by hematoxylin and eosin, periodic acid-Schiff, periodic acid-Schiff following diastase, Masson trichrome, reticulin stain, van Gieson elastica method, and Perls' iron stain. Direct immunofluorescence staining for immunoglobulins (IgG, IgM, IgA), complement, and fibrinogen was performed on frozen sections in four cases (case 2, 5, 6 and 7). For detection of antibasement membrane antibody, sera from patients with IPH (cases 2, 5, 6 and 7) were tested by indirect immunofluorescence against normal human or rat lung and kidney [16]. Electron microscopic examination was performed on lung biopsies from cases 2, 5, 6 and 7.

Pathology

The histopathologic abnormalities in our cases of IPH were in general agreement with those described in the literature [6, 17], and the findings were evaluated semiquantitatively (table III).

The lung biopsy from a patient who later died after massive hemoptysis (case 1) showed extensive interstitial fibrosis, hyperplasia of type II alveolar epithelial cells, and clusters of hemosiderin-containing macrophages and red cells in the alveolar spaces. The lung at autopsy was similar except for more extensive recent hemorrhage and dilatation of small pulmonary vessels. Pulmonary hilar lymph nodes, but not other organs, con-

---

Fig. 1a, b. Lung biopsy in case 2. *a* Low magnification view of lung periphery showing some alveolar spaces filled with numerous hemosiderin-laden macrophages (arrow-head) whereas others show recent hemorrhage and edema (asterix). In this area, the alveolar septa appear relatively normal. HE. ×160. *b* An alveolar septum lined by cuboidal type II cells with vacuolated cytoplasm. Except for slight increase in type II cells no other abnormality is apparent. The alveoli contain small pools of red cells (arrows) and clusters of alveolar macrophages (AM). 1-μm section. Toluidine blue. ×640.

Fig. 2a, b. Lung biopsy in case 3. *a* Low magnification view showing an area of lung consolidation due to interstitial fibrosis and filling of alveoli with hemosiderin-laden macrophages. Lumen of a small bronchiole (Br) also contains clusters of hemosiderin-filled macrophages. Perls' Prussian blue stain. ×70. *b* Close-up view from figure 2a, showing massive accumulation of hemosiderin in the cytoplasm of macrophages within the alveoli (Alv), septal macrophages, and connective tissue (arrows). Perls' Prussian blue stain. ×640.

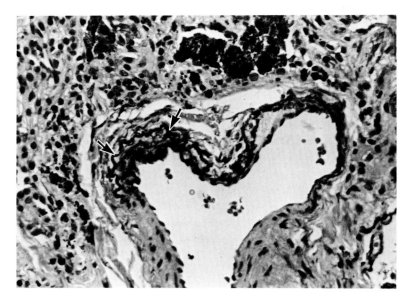

Fig. 3. Part of a wall of a small pulmonary artery in a lung biopsy (case 5) with encrustation of elastic laminae by hemosiderin (arrows). Hemosiderin granules are also seen in interstitial macrophages and free in connective tissue (top). HE and Perls' Prussian blue stain. ×640.

tained hemosiderin and there was no evidence of renal or collagen-vascular disease.

The extent of involvement in lung biopsies varied. Most specimens contained areas of consolidation, due to massive accumulation of hemosiderin-laden macrophages with obliteration of alveolar spaces and interstitial fibrosis, alternating with areas of relatively normal lung parenchyma (fig. 1a). The amount of recent hemorrhage varied from occasional red cells in a few alveoli to complete filling of alveolar spaces with fresh blood (fig. 1b), and it was difficult to evaluate because of the possible contribution of surgical trauma. Alveolar edema was occasionally present in addition to recent hemorrhage. Stainable iron, finely to coarsly granular was localized predominantly in alveolar macrophages (fig. 2a, b). Focal iron deposits in the interstitium were either in macrophages or free in connective tissue (fig. 2b). In three cases (case 1, 3 and 5), the elastic fibers of small blood vessels and alveolar septa were focally encrusted with iron

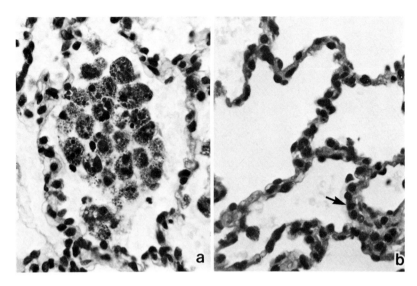

Fig. 4a, b. Lung biopsy (case 2). *a* Increased number of cuboidal, alveolar type II cells lining an alveolus partially filled with hemosiderin-laden macrophages. The alveolar septa show no evidence of fibrosis or cellular infiltrate. HE. ×640. *b* Another area of lung from the same sample (as in a) without hemorrhage or hemosiderin containing macrophages in alveoli showing prominence of alveolar type II cells (arrows). HE. ×640.

and calcium (fig. 3). All cases had mild to moderate hyperplasia of alveolar type II cells. The number of cuboidal type II cells appeared increased regardless of whether the alveoli were filled with hemosiderin-containing macrophages (fig. 4a, b). The alveolar septa were generally thicker in areas of massive iron deposition (fig. 2a), with fibrosis and chronic inflammatory cell infiltrates. Both the consolidated and the 'normal' areas of lung contained focal peribronchial aggregates of lymphoid tissue. Acute inflammatory cells, including eosinophils, were rare but all specimens contained a marked increase in mast cells, particularly within alveolar septa, close to small blood vessels.

Immunopathology
Immunofluorescence of biopsy specimens was negative for immunoglobulins and complement, and antibasement membrane antibodies could not be identified in serum samples as in other reported studies [12, 14, 15].

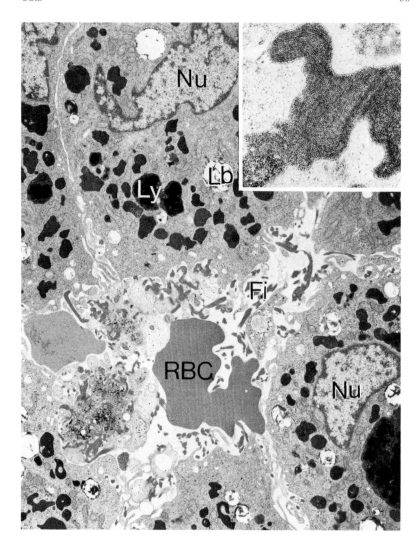

Fig. 5. Electron micrograph of alveolar macrophages clustered around red cells (RBC) and fibrin (Fi), indicating recent intra-alveolar hemorrhage. The macrophages have eccentrically placed nuclei (Nu) and their cytoplasm contains numerous lysosomes (Ly) filled with hemosiderin pigment and occasional phagocytosed lamellar bodies (Lb) originating from alveolar type II cells (case 2, lung biopsy). TEM. ×6,500. Insert: Higher magnification of a pleomorphic lysosome with crystalline arrays representing ferritin particles. TEM. ×44,000.

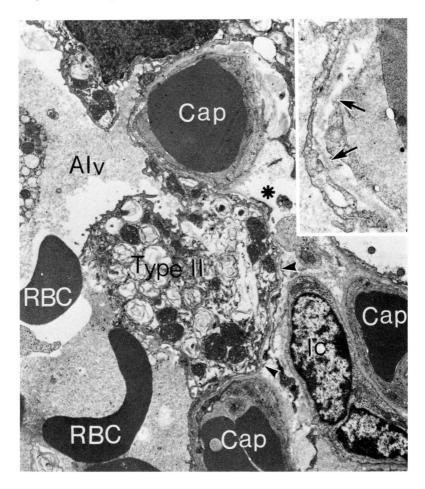

Fig. 6. Electron micrograph of an alveolar septum showing parts of three alveolar capillaries (Cap) in an area of recent hemorrhage. The alveolar lumen (Alv) contains red blood cells (RBC) and flocculent proteinaceous edema fluid. The cytoplasm of alveolar type II cells shows focal degenerative changes and large electron dense mitochondria. The alveolar basement membrane (arrow heads) appears intact. Focal interstitial edema (asterisk) and normal interstitial cells (Ic) between two alveolar capillaries (case 2, lung biopsy). TEM. ×6,500. Insert: Higher magnification of thin portion of alveolar capillary membrane with focal discontinuity of basement membrane (arrows). TEM. ×28,000.

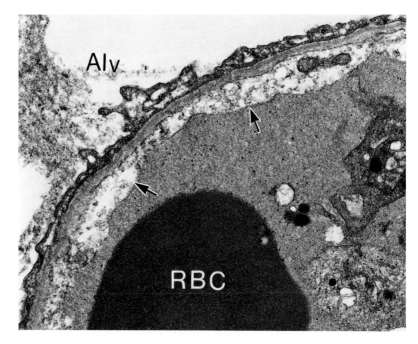

Fig. 7. Air-blood barrier in another area of recent intra-alveolar hemorrhage with focal swelling of endothelial cell cytoplasm (arrows). The surface of alveolar type I cell shows prominent irregular microvilli and cytoplasmic invaginations. The fused portion of alveolar basement membrane appears well preserved. Alveolar lumen (Alv) contains some edema fluid (case 2, lung biopsy). TEM. ×21,000.

Electron Microscopy

Electron microscopic examination of four specimens (table III) showed electron-dense, membrane-bound inclusions typical of hemosiderin within macrophages (fig. 5). The inclusions were homogeneous to finely granular, with crystalline-like arrangement (fig. 5, insert). Macrophages also contained phagocytosed concentric lamellar bodies originating from type II cells. Fragments of red cells and fibrin lay among the macrophages, indicating recent hemorrhage (fig. 5).

Focal degeneration and shedding of alveolar type II cells were present in areas of severe recent alveolar hemorrhage and edema (fig. 6). Although the type I cells generally appeared normal, their cytoplasmic processes covering the thin portions of alveolar capillary walls formed irregular microvillous projections with deep invaginations; the cytoplasm of endothelial cells was focally swollen (fig. 7). The basal laminae in the

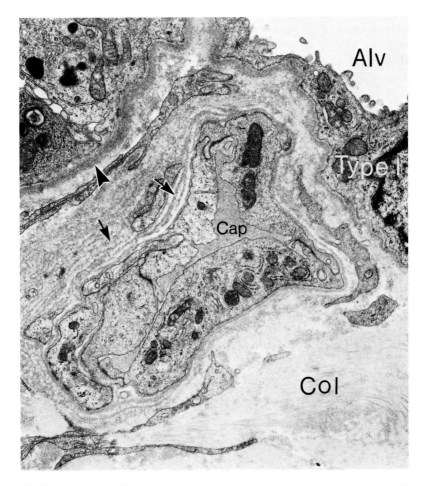

Fig. 8. Prominent multilayering of basement membrane (arrows) around a septal capillary (Cap). Alveolar basement membrane appears focally thickened (arrowhead) compared to an area covered with alveolar type I cells. Col=Collagen (case 6, lung biopsy). TEM. ×13,500.

fused portions of alveolar capillary basement membranes appeared slightly thickened, with focal discontinuities in the lamina densa (fig. 6, insert). However complete breaks and immune complex deposits were not observed in any of the samples examined. In one case, reduplication of the basal lamina with an onion skin-like arrangement was seen around the deeper septal capillaries (fig. 8).

Although the increased number of alveolar type II cells, noted by

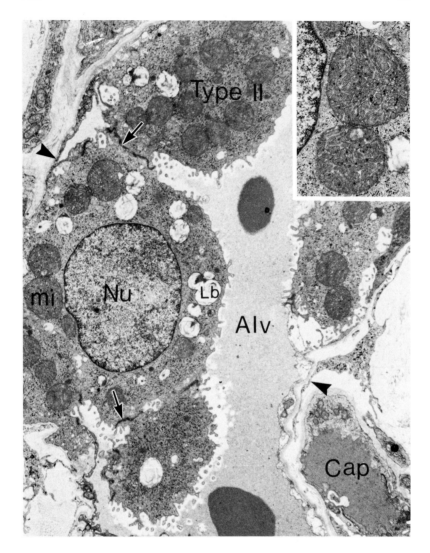

Fig. 9. Part of an 'intact' alveolar wall with increased number of type II cells. These cells have prominent microvilli on the apex and tight junctions between lateral surfaces (arrows). The cytoplasm contains a vesicular nucleus (Nu), numerous abnormally large mitochondria, and characteristic lamellar bodies (LB). The basement membrane (arrow heads) shows no abnormalities. The alveolar lumen (Alv) contains some edema fluid but no hemosiderin-laden macrophages. TEM. ×6,500. Insert: High magnification of type II cell mitochondria with closely packed tubular cristae and increased number of dense bodies (case 2, lung biopsy). TEM. ×15,500.

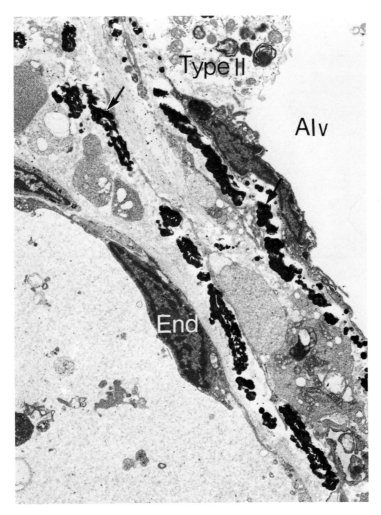

Fig. 10. Massive dark mineral deposits (iron-calcium phosphate) within interstitium (arrows). Type I and II cells lining the alveolus (Alv) show focal degenerative changes, whereas endothelial cells (End) of a septal lymphatic appear normal (case 5, lung biopsy). TEM. ×7,600.

light microscopy and confirmed by electron microscopy, is commonly regarded as a nonspecific reaction of the lung to injury, we observed hyperplasia of type II cells in both involved and 'normal' areas (fig. 9). The hyperplastic type II cells also exhibited several unusual features including an increased number of free ribosomes, prominent Golgi com-

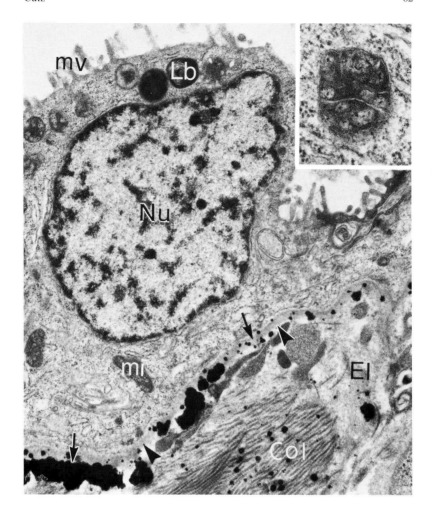

Fig. 11. Electron-dense mineral deposits (arrows) within and under alveolar basement membrane (arrowheads). Small granular deposits are also seen in elastic fibers (El) and collagen (Col). Adjacent type II cells show sparse surface microvilli (mv), few lamellar bodies (Lb) and mitochondria (mi) with dense matrix. The nucleus (Nu) appears normal (case 5, lung biopsy). TEM. ×14,800. Insert: Close-up of a mitochondrion with electron-dense matrix and distorted cristae containing irregular dense deposits (? ferruginous bodies). TEM. ×44,000.

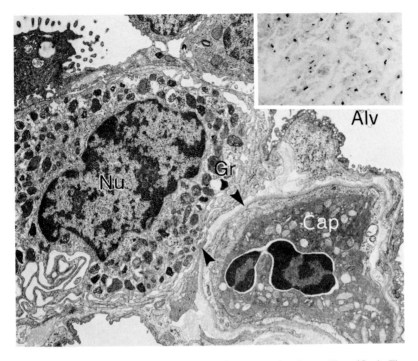

Fig. 12. A mast cell within alveolar septum close to an alveolar capillary (Cap). The mast cell contains a centrally placed nucleus (Nu), typical cytoplasmic granules (Gr) and is in close contact with capillary basement membrane (arrowheads). Polymorph (PMN) is present within the capillary lumen (case 6, lung biopsy). TEM. ×9,800. Insert: Large number of mast cells scattered within alveolar septae in a relatively 'normal' area of lung (case 6). Aldehyde fuchsin stain. ×160.

plexes, and enlarged mitochondria with closely packed, somewhat distorted cristae and numerous dense bodies (fig. 9, insert). The size, number and appearance of cytoplasmic lamellar inclusions were normal.

Electron microscopic examination (case 5) has shown mineralization of the elastic fibers by iron and calcium to take the form of particulate, extremely electron dense deposits in the elastic laminae of blood vessels and the elastic fibers of the alveolar septa (fig. 10). Similar but smaller deposits were also found in association with collagen fibres and focally within the capillary basement membranes (fig. 11). Mitochondria of type II alveolar epithelial cells contained disorganized cristae and irregular dense bodies resembling the ferruginous deposits described in immature normoblasts (fig. 11, insert).

The alveolar septa contained occasional macrophages with hemo-siderin granules and numerous mast cells (fig. 12). Two types of mast cells were identified, one containing granules with tubular, scroll-like inclusions and, in the other, granules with particulate floccular densities. In several instances the mast cells were located within the alveolar septa, with little or no connective tissue separating them from the alveolar capil-laries.

Pulmonary Hemosiderosis (PH) Associated with Sensitivity to Cow's Milk

In 1962 Heiner et al. [18] reported PH associated with sensitivity to cow's milk in seven infants and children with recurrent respiratory disease, chronic rhinitis, recurrent otitis media, growth retardation, high titers of precipitin antibodies, and positive skin tests to cow's milk proteins. Four patients (all young infants) had clinical and laboratory findings of 'idiopathic pulmonary hemosiderosis.' The symptoms improved when cow's milk was removed from the diet and recurred upon its reintroduc-tion. Boat et al. [19] have since described a group of infants and young children with high titers of milk precipitin and PH, and with cor pulmonale secondary to nasopharyngeal obstruction. As in the cases of Heiner et al. [18], elimination of cow's milk from the diet and adenoidectomy (when in-dicated) resulted in clinical improvement. It has been suggested, there-fore, that sensitivity to cow's milk may be causally related to PH. How-ever, the significance of milk precipitin in PH and respiratory disorders in general remains controversial, and the precise immunologic mechanisms have not been defined. Immunofluorescence studies on lung biopsies from two patients with cow's milk-induced PH have shown granular deposits of IgG, IgA, C3, fibrinogen, and bovine serum albumin diffusely scattered throughout the lung parenchyma and in polymorphonuclear leukocytes [20], and immune complex deposition or an Arthus-like phenomenon has been proposed to be the underlying mechanism. Although some patients have elevation of serum IgE concentration or specific IgE antibodies against alpha-casein and bovine serum albumin [21], it is uncertain whether these findings relate directly to the pathogenesis of PH. In a de-tailed immunologic study of patients with cow's milk-induced PH, no specific defect involving either humoral or cellular immunity could be demonstrated [16].

The patients with cow's milk-induced PH differ in many respects from those with typical IPH. They are younger (the first symptoms usually develop prior to 6 months of age), there is an apparent predominance of black infants, and most patients have a variety of other respiratory symptoms attributable to allergy [19]. Only about 10% of patients with pulmonary manifestations related to cow's milk sensitivity develop PH, and elevated precipitin to cow's milk protein can be also found in asymptomatic children [20, 21]. Older patients with IPH (including those in the present study) have neither evidence of milk allergy nor dramatic symptomatic improvement while consuming milk-free diets [2]. Although the significance of sensitivity to cow's milk proteins remains unclear, this syndrome should be considered in the differential diagnosis of pulmonary hemorrhage and hemosiderosis, particularly in young infants.

Pulmonary Hemorrhage and Glomerulonephritis

The association of pulmonary hemorrhage and glomerulonephritis, now commonly referred to as Goodpasture's syndrome (GS), was first reported in 1919 by Goodpasture [22] in the case of a young male patient who died during an influenza epidemic. Immunopathological and experimental studies during the last two decades have defined this syndrome as a type II or cytotoxic antibody-mediated reaction characterized by antibodies directed against glomerular (GBM) and alveolar basement membrane [23]. With increasing awareness and wider application of immunologic techniques, it became apparent that the combination of pulmonary hemorrhage and glomerulonephritis can occur without detectable GBM antibodies in patients who may exhibit other immune reactions. Because of basic pathogenetic differences with implications for treatment and prognosis, the diagnosis of Goodpasture's syndrome (or more correctly anti-GBM disease) has been restricted to patients with demonstrable GBM antibodies. Since pulmonary hemorrhage is frequently the initial presenting symptom, these two disorders are important considerations in the differential diagnosis of IPH. The following discussion will be focused mainly on the conditions in infants and children.

Goodpasture's Syndrome

In contrast to IPH, GS is reported to occur primarily in young Caucasian males in their twenties [24]. However, in a recent series of 29 patients reported from New Zealand, the ages ranged from 17 to 68 years and one-third of the patients were females [25]. There are only a few case reports of GS in children under 10 years of age [26, 27], with only one well-documented case with GBM antibodies [28]. The files of The Hospital for Sick Children for the last 25 years contains a single case of possible GS in a 2.5-year-old girl who presented at 10 months of age with severe iron deficiency anemia, pulmonary infiltrates and hemoptysis. After initial improvement, she developed several exacerbations that included pulmonary symptoms as well as hematuria and proteinuria. She died of massive pulmonary hemorrhage and autopsy showed acute pulmonary hemorrhage with extensive hemosiderosis and fibrosis. The kidneys showed crescentic glomerulonephritis with focal hyalinization. Immunohistochemical and electron microscopic studies were not performed, precluding a definitive diagnosis of GS. Most patients with GS present first with pulmonary hemorrhage, followed weeks or months later by renal disease. The clinical course is typically stormy and characterized by rapid deterioration and, until recently, almost invariably fatal outcome [29]. The cause of death is usually due to massive hemoptysis or acute renal failure. In milder cases the clinical symptoms resemble those of IPH, with hemoptysis, dyspnea, and iron-deficiency anemia. The radiologic, pulmonary function and laboratory findings may be indistinguishable for IPH. The renal disease, which may be silent for extended periods of time, may vary from mild to severe glomerulonephritis, with proteinuria and variable hematuria [29].

The histopathologic changes in the lung resemble those seen in patients with IPH and include both recent and old intra-alveolar hemorrhage with numerous hemosiderin-laden macrophages [24, 25, 30]. The renal changes in a florid stage are usually those of rapidly progressive glomerulonephritis, with extensive crescent formation, necrosis of glomerular tufts, and focal obliteration of glomeruli [31]. The hallmark of GS is the uniformly linear deposition of IgG (less commonly IgM or IgA) along the glomerular and alveolar basement membranes [24, 25, 31]. Positive staining for complement is demonstrable in about 75% of specimens and is distributed in focal segmental or sometimes granular pattern [31]. Mixed linear and granular (immune-complex type) immune staining patterns in glomeruli [32, 33] and evolution of a granular into a linear staining pattern have been reported [34]. It is unclear whether such cases represent variants of GS or coexistence of two disease processes with different immunologic mechanisms.

Ultrastructural studies of kidney biopsies have revealed a variety of glomerular changes, none of which appears to be specific for GBM-induced injury [31]. The most frequently reported changes in GBM include widening of the subendothelial lucent zones (laminae rarae) and a diffuse increase in the density in the laminae densae [35]. Electron-dense deposits, as commonly seen in immune complex glomerulonephritis, are invariably absent. Disruption of GBM occurs as in other types of crescentic glomerulonephritis [31].

Information about ultrastructural changes in the alveolar capillary walls is scanty. Donald et al. [36] found evidence of diffuse vascular injury, i.e. wide endothelial gaps, diffuse fragmentation, and increased electron density of alveolar capillary basement membrane in a lung biopsy from one patient with GS. In contrast, they did not find similar changes in lung biopsies from three patients with IPH. Teague et al. [25] observed hyperplasia of type II pneumocytes and variation in the width and electron density of the alveolar basement membrane in lung biopsy specimens from three patients with GS.

Because the lesions observed in both kidney and lung relate to GBM antibodies and because the majority of patients with GS have circulating GBM antibodies [37], the role of GBM antibodies in the pathogenesis of GS appears to be well established. Antibodies eluted from glomeruli cross-react with alveolar and glomerular basement membrane antigens explaining the concurrent involvement of both lung and kidney [38]. Experimental studies demonstrate lesions similar to those of GS following injection of basement membrane antigens or eluates of kidney or lung tissue from affected patients [39].

The etiology and factors promoting the formation of GBM antibodies remain obscure. Some studies suggested that the initial insult involves the lung, whereby viral infection [40] or exposure to toxic hydrocarbon fumes [41] triggers the release of basement membrane antigens. Genetic predisposition to GS is suggested by occasional reports of familial cases and by an apparent association with HLA group, DRW2 [42, 43].

Pulmonary Hemorrhage and Glomerulonephritis without
GBM Antibodies

Several patients are reported to have had a clinical picture indistinguishable from GS, but without demonstrable GBM antibodies or evidence of multisystem collagen-vascular disease. Most of them have had an immune-complex glomerulonephritis. A single case of pulmonary hemosiderosis in association with asymptomatic IgA nephropathy occurred in a 17-year-old boy [44]. Loughlin et al. [45] reported 2 girls, aged 8 and 11

years who had anemia, hemoptysis, renal failure and crescentic glomerulonephritis highly suggestive of GS, but without GBM antibodies or positive serologic tests for collagen-vascular disease. Immunofluorescence revealed coarse, granular deposits of IgG, IgM and C3 in glomerular capillary walls and mesangial areas. A lung biopsy from one of the patients
showed recent and old intra-alveolar hemorrhage with numerous hemosiderin-laden macrophages and no immune-complex deposits or vasculitis.
The authors concluded that their patients had an idiopathic immune-complex nephritis associated with pulmonary hemorrhage, and they emphasized the need for detailed immunologic and immunopathologic studies to
differentiate this disorder from GS and other pulmonary-renal syndromes.
Long-term follow-up may be required to rule out the possibility that these
patients have variants of GS [32–34] or early stages of collagen-vascular
disease, such as SLE (see next section).

Pulmonary hemorrhage and renal failure reported in patients with
Wilson's disease receiving D-penicillamine [46] probably represent drug-
induced immune-complex disease, as no GBM antibodies have been detected and immunofluorescence has shown a granular pattern of staining.

Pulmonary Hemosiderosis Associated with Systemic Collagen Vascular or Purpuric Disease

Acute pulmonary hemorrhage and hemosiderosis are rare but well-
recognized features of systemic collagen-vascular disease and various purpuric disorders. These two broad disease categories are discussed together
because of many overlapping clinical and laboratory findings [29, 31].
These disorders may be difficult to differentiate from IPH, particularly
when pulmonary symptoms develop prior to systemic manifestations.

Diffuse pulmonary hemorrhage is a relatively uncommon initial manifestation in systemic lupus erythematosis (SLE) [47, 48], and it may pre-
cede by months or years the development of classical clinical features [49,
50]. Pulmonary hemorrhage in SLE, with or without renal involvement,
affects mostly adults, occasionally children younger than 10 years [51]. Although the initial clinical and radiologic features of lung hemorrhage in
SLE may closely resemble those of IPH, a positive antinuclear antibody
test, LE cells, hypocomplementemia and other serologic tests will establish the diagnosis of SLE.

The light microscopic findings in lung biopsies and autopsy samples include diffuse intra-alveolar hemorrhage filling the alveoli with red cells and hemosiderin-laden macrophages, and often there are also changes of diffuse alveolar damage [49]. Findings that may implicate SLE in the differential diagnosis include cellular subintimal proliferation and organized intramural thrombi in the small blood vessels, although florid vasculitis and fibrinoid necrosis are uncommon [49].

The basic pathogenic mechanism responsible for pulmonary hemorrhage in SLE is deposition of immune complexes in the lung. Some patients with SLE may have additional factors such as pulmonary infection, bleeding diathesis, and 'shock lung' syndrome. The alveolar septa, walls of larger blood vessels, and bronchioles contain typical granular deposits of IgG, IgM and complement; no immune complex deposits were observed in patients with SLE and pulmonary disease without alveolar hemorrhage [49]. Subendothelial electron dense deposits, sometimes with a 'fingerprint' pattern identical to that seen in the kidney, have been demonstrated within the alveolar capillary basement membranes [50, 52]. The other ultrastructural findings included diffuse alveolar and endothelial cell injury [49].

In disorders characterized by systemic vasculitis, such as Wegener's granulomatosis, periarteritis nodosa, and rheumatoid arthritis, the pulmonary vessels may be involved, leading to diffuse pulmonary hemorrhage [2, 3, 29–31, 53]. These disorders rarely affect children and are more common in adults. With typical clinical and pathologic features of systemic vasculitis, the differentiation from IPH is usually not a problem, although there can be a confusing clinical and pathological picture [53]. O'Donohue [54] reported an 18-year-old female patient who initially was thought to have IPH, but she developed over a period of 2 years the clinical features and positive serologic tests suggestive of several connective tissue disorders. Later in her course she developed cavitary pulmonary nodules, vasculitic skin lesions, and nasal involvement indicative of Wegener's granulomatosis. Schachter et al. [55] reported a similar case.

Systemic vasculitis associated with pulmonary hemorrhage is rare in patients younger than 10 years. Cunningham and Hammond [56] reported a case of a 5-year-old girl with pulmonary hemosiderosis and an undefined collagen vascular syndrome manifested at autopsy by arteritis involving multiple organs, pericarditis, myocarditis, glomerulonephritis, and arthritis. Perelman et al. [57] described a 3-year-old girl with pulmonary hemosiderosis and clinical and laboratory features of both SLE and rheumatoid arthritis.

Pulmonary hemorrhage is a rare manifestation of purpuric disorders, including Schönlein-Henoch purpura [53, 58] and idiopathic thrombocytopenic purpura [2]. A previously unreported association of microangiopathic hemolytic anemia with pulmonary vasculitis has been described in adults [3]. A 7-year-old girl with initial clinical and laboratory findings suggestive of IPH had marked thrombocytopenia and antiplatelet antibodies [59]. A good clinical response to corticosteroid treatment and splenectomy suggested idiopathic thrombocytopenic purpura, but she subsequently developed a fatal, poorly defined connective tissue disorder with systemic vasculitis.

Pulmonary Hemosiderosis Secondary to Cardiac Disease, Intrapulmonary Vascular Lesions or Malformations

As hemosiderin-containing macrophages in the lung are common in patients with heart disease, an underlying cardiac abnormality should be included in the differential diagnosis of pulmonary hemosiderosis. The pathophysiology of pulmonary hemorrhage secondary to cardiac disease relates to increased pulmonary venous and capillary pressure with diapedesis of red cells into the alveoli. Any cardiac lesion associated with increased pulmonary venous pressure may cause pulmonary hemorrhage and subsequent deposition of hemosiderin pigment. The commonest cardiac abnormalities associated with pulmonary hemosiderosis are mitral stenosis and chronic left- or right-sided heart failure [2, 60].

Pulmonary hemosiderosis is a common feature of pulmonary hypertension, particularly when advanced vascular changes are present [61]. A combination of increased pressure and intrinsic vascular lesions contribute to pathogenesis of pulmonary hemorrhage.

Acute pulmonary hemorrhage can complicate intrapulmonary arteriovenous fistulas and other congenital vascular malformations [62], pulmonary venoocclusive disease [63], and pulmonary lymphangioleiomyomatosis, in young women [64]. The diagnosis of these lesions, particularly pulmonary venoocclusive disease could be missed on small lung biopsy specimens unless elastic tissue stains are performed.

Pulmonary vascular thrombosis, as seen in patients with sickle cell disease and nephrotic syndrome may lead to pulmonary hemosiderosis. In a resolving stage, this lesion may be confused with IPH.

Other Associations

Pulmonary hemosiderosis and pulmonary hemorrhage occur in association with different disease processes [2, 3, 29–31] that may be related causally or coincidentally. For the association between pulmonary hemosiderosis and celiac disease in both adults [65] and children [66] an immunologic mechanism has been proposed but not proven. Morgan and Turner-Warwick [3] reported 2 adults with diabetes mellitus, acute pulmonary hemorrhage and renal failure. Electron microscopy of lung biopsies revealed marked changes in alveolar capillary basement membrane and endothelium. While such changes may predispose to pulmonary hemorrhage, they can be present in other tissues of diabetic patients with no evidence of local hemorrhage.

Exposure to drugs and toxins may also lead to acute pulmonary hemorrhage. A Goodpasture's-like syndrome has been reported in patients with Wilson's disease treated with D-penicillamine (see p. 68). Hemolytic anemia and repeated episodes of hemoptysis have been described in 2 young men exposed to epoxy resin containing trimellitic anhydride [67]. Antibodies against trimellitic anhydride suggested an immunologic mechanism. The symptoms resolved spontaneously when the patients were no longer exposed to the toxin.

Pathogenesis and Pathophysiology

The pathogenetic mechanisms of intrapulmonary hemorrhage include direct damage to the pulmonary vasculature, e.g. vasculitis, deposition of antibodies or immune complexes, congenital and acquired abnormalities of pulmonary blood vessels, increased pressure in the pulmonary circulation, and hematologic disorders (table IV). These factors and mechanisms may be involved singly or in combination.

IPH is by definition a disease of unknown etiology, and the pathogenesis of repeated intrapulmonary hemorrhage remains unknown. Specific infectious agents and toxic substances have not been implicated, and immunologic studies have not identified immune complexes or antibodies to substantiate an immunologic mechanism of injury [12, 14, 15]. A few reports of familial IPH suggest that genetic factors play a role [8, 9], but the majority of cases appear to be sporadic.

IPH has been hypothesized to result from a primary structural defect

Table IV. Pathogenesis and mechanisms of diffuse PH

Disease entity	Mechanism or basic defect	
	defined	presumed or proposed
Idiopathic pulmonary hemosiderosis		abnormal elastica [5] defect in alveolar lining cells [6,17] abnormal alveolar capillary b.m. [14, 15, 36, 68, 69]
PH associated with hyper-sensitivity to cow's milk		immune complexes [20, 21] Arthus-like reaction [20, 21] immediate-type hyper-sensitivity [20, 21]
Goodpasture's syndrome	antibasement membrane antibody [23]	
PH and glomerulonephritis (without GBM antibodies)	immune complexes [45]	
Systemic lupus erythematosus	immune complexes [49]	
Wegener's granulomatosis	vasculitis [53–55]	
Polyarteritis nodosa	vasculitis [29–31, 53]	
Rheumatoid arthritis	vasculitis [2, 29–31]	
Idiopathic thrombo-cytopenic purpura	bleeding diathesis, anti-platelet antibodies± vasculitis [2, 59]	
PH secondary to cardiac disease or intrapulmonary vascular abnormality	↑ pulmonary venous pressure and/or pulmonary vascular lesions [2, 61, 62]	
PH associated with celiac disease		? immunologic mechanisms [65]
PH associated with D-penicillamine treatment	immune complexes [46]	
PH associated with trimellitic anhydride	antibodies against serum albumin and red cells [67]	

in the pulmonary microcirculation with an inherent 'weakness' of capillary walls. Evidence from chest radiographs and from histologic appearances suggests that the bleeding in IPH is multifocal, and occurs in the lung periphery at the level of small airways and alveoli [3, 6, 17]. Early histopathologic studies, prior to the advent of electron microscopy, suggested an abnormal development of elastic fibers in the pulmonary vessels as the primary defect in IPH [5]. Although this possibility retains some consideration, it has no direct evidence in its support. The changes in elastic fibers (e.g. fragmentation and encrustation with iron and calcium) are considered now to be secondary to interstitial deposition of hemosiderin. Soergel and Sommers [6, 17], who reported the largest series of IPH with detailed light microscopic study, described abnormally tortuous and dilated alveolar capillaries and suggested that they may be the sites of pulmonary bleeding. These vascular changes, however, are seen most commonly in fatal cases and are likely to be the result of terminal heart failure and pulmonary congestion.

Electron microscopy has clarified many aspects of normal and abnormal lung structure, particularly those related to the air-blood barrier. Unfortunately, ultrastructural studies have failed to reveal the basic defect of IPH. Discrepancies among the reported studies could reflect differences in the ages of the patients (more than half of the cases studied were adults), in activity of the disease process, or in the focal nature of the lesions, and most studies were based on single cases.

Whereas some EM studies of lung biopsies in IPH have shown intact alveolar capillary walls [12], others showed abnormalities in the capillary basement membrane such as focal splitting, increased collagen deposition or diffuse thickening and reduplication [14, 15, 68]. Most of these changes are probably nonspecific as they accompany many types of alveolar injury [30]. Deposits of iron and calcium in the vessel walls and close to the alveolar basement membrane could increase fragility of those structures and perpetuate episodes of hemorrhage [69], but these changes are clearly secondary to interstitial hemorrhage and the trapping of hemosiderin.

Focal breaks in otherwise normal alveolar capillary walls were reported by Hyatt et al. [70], but not confirmed by others. Donald et al. demonstrated extravasation of red cells in areas with disruption of an abnormally thickened and 'smudged' alveolar capillary basement membranes [36]. We have observed focal discontinuity of the lamina densa but only in areas of recent hemorrhage, which, with changes in alveolar type I cells and endothelial cells, would be consistent with recent injury and extravasation at that site. Whether such lesions are primary or secondary is difficult to answer from static morphologic studies.

It is not surprising that open defects in basement membrane are demonstrated only infrequently if one considers the focal nature of these lesions and the problem of sampling for electron microscopic examination, a situation paralleling the study of glomerular disease associated with hematuria. In an extensive study of the glomerular basement membrane in a variety of renal diseases, gaps and breaks were observed only in cases with most severe lesions (e.g. necrosis of capillary walls, massive intramembranous deposits, and polymorphonuclear infiltrates) and only after considerable search on a large number of sections [71]. Furthermore, gaps in the basement membrane are often covered by cytoplasmic processes of epithelial or endothelial cells, indicating a rapid cellular response with sealing of the leak.

Most previous EM studies in IPH have focused on the status of alveolar capillary basement membrane, with little attention to cellular components of the alveolar wall. The involvement of alveolar epithelial cells in the pathogenesis of IPH has been suggested by Soergel and Sommers, who observed diffuse hyperplasia of alveolar lining cells with focal areas of degeneration and shedding, irrespective of the duration of the disease or presence of intra-alveolar hemorrhage [17]. Our findings are in agreement with this observation. The ultrastructural abnormalities of the alveolar type II cells, known to play an important role in the production of surfactant and to be progenitor cells of alveolar type I cells [72], suggests that dysfunction of these cells leads to derangement of alveolar stability and of the air-blood barrier. Changes in type II cell mitochondria included increased size and number and abnormally arranged cristae, although further studies are needed to determine if these changes represent an intrinsic mitochondrial abnormality, specific for IPH, or a reactive phenomenon. We have not seen similar mitochondrial changes in other pulmonary disorders characterized by type II cell hyperplasia, such as desquamative interstitial pneumonitis, viral pneumonitis, and oxygen toxicity [73]. Furthermore, pulmonary hemorrhage associated with immunologically mediated renal disease has not been associated with mitochondrial abnormalities in alveolar type II cells [36].

Numerous mast cells were concentrated within the alveolar septa. Although increased number of mast cells in the lung is found in a variety of pulmonary disorders (e.g. pulmonary fibrosis and asthma), the mast cells are usually concentrated around the airways and large blood vessels and in areas of fibrosis [74, 75]. In contrast, mast cells in IPH were increased even in areas without interstitial fibrosis and appeared in close proximity to pulmonary microvasculature. The presence of mast cells at this strategic location may be of pathophysiological significance, because release of bioactive substances may affect the vascular tonus and permeability [76]. Activation of mast cells to release mediators is usually, but not always, immunologically mediated [77]. Except for possible association of pulmonary hemosiderosis with allergy to milk proteins, there is no evidence of an immediate-type hypersensitivity reaction in IPH, and further studies are required to determine the role of mast cells in the pathophysiology of IPH and related disorders.

The main consequences of repeated intrapulmonary hemorrhage are chronic blood loss and deposition of hemosiderin pigment. An iron-deficiency anemia in these patients is aggravated by sequestration of iron in alveolar macrophages, making iron molecules inaccessible for metabolism. Accumulation of hemosiderin, an iron containing by-product of hemoglobin breakdown [78] in alveolar macrophages and to a certain extent in the lung interstitium is thought to be responsible for the development of pulmonary fibrosis and chronic lung disease. However, this may be an oversimplification, and other factors and mechanisms may be involved. Recent studies of iron metabolism suggest that the cellular site of iron overload is the important determinant of cell and tissue damage and of progression of the disease process [79]. For example, fibrosis or cirrhosis is more common in liver disorders associated with significant iron overload in hepatocytes as opposed to those conditions in which Kupffer cells are the main storage site. Removal of excess iron by treatment with chelating agents is beneficial in some conditions with iron overload [80], but this approach has not been used extensively in the treatment of IPH and related disorders.

Concluding Remarks

Diffuse pulmonary hemorrhage and hemosiderosis is a rare clinical and pathological manifestation of a variety of disease processes. Idiopathic pulmonary hemosiderosis, characterized by intrapulmonary bleeding without an apparent cause, is the most common and also the most problematic form of the disorder usually affecting children under 10 years of age. The diagnosis of IPH is restricted to patients in whom detailed clinical and laboratory investigation, including immunologic studies and a lung biopsy, have ruled out all other known causes of intrapulmonary hemorrhage. Apart from cases in which pulmonary hemorrhage is associated with cardiac disease, intrapulmonary vascular abnormality or a hematologic disorder, the most important conditions in the differential diagnosis of IPH are the pulmonary-renal syndromes and collagen vascular-diseases. While the latter are more common in adults, they can also occur in children. In many such cases, the initial clinical presentation may be confusing and often mimic IPH. Long-term follow-up of patients is required to establish the diagnosis.

Detailed ultrastructural and immunopathologic studies of lung and kidney biopsy specimens should be performed in every patient presenting with diffuse pulmonary hemorrhage. Of importance is the identification of underlying immunologic mechanisms and the differentiation between disorders mediated by antibasement membrane antibodies (Goodpasture's syndrome) and those conditions in which vascular damage is induced by immune complexes. Immunologic mechanisms appear to be involved in pulmonary hemorrhage associated with drug treatment (e.g. penicillamine in Wilson's disease), exposure to toxins (e.g. trimellitic anhydride) and possibly celiac disease. The causal relationship between pulmonary hemorrhage and allergy to milk proteins is uncertain, it seems to be restricted to young infants with allergic symptoms in other organ systems. There is no direct evidence that immunologic mechanisms play a role in the pathogenesis of IPH.

Although the etiology and pathogenesis of IPH are unknown, the disease process is restricted to the lung and it is localized at the level of alveolar capillary membrane. The presumed defect is thought to be an abnormality of alveolar air-blood barrier involving either the basement membrane or alveolar lining cells, but the nature of the defect and whether it is primary or acquired remains undefined. Future investigation should focus on the structure-function correlation of the air-blood barrier [81], biochemistry and metabolism of basement membrane material [82], biology and pathophysiology of alveolar lining cells [83] and the control of pulmonary microcirculation [84].

Acknowledgements

The author thanks his clinical colleagues Drs. J.A.P. Turner and H. Levison for reviewing the manuscript and for their helpful suggestions. Thanks are also due to Veronica Wong for technical assistance in preparing electron micrographs, to Michael Starr for preparation of photographs and to Anne Warner for typing the manuscript.

References

1 Thomas, H.M.; Irwin, R.S.: Classification of diffuse intrapulmonary hemorrhage. Chest *68:* 483 (1975).

2 Heiner, D.C.: Pulmonary hemosiderosis; in Kendig, Chernick, Disorders of the respiratory tract in children, pp. 538–552 (Saunders, Philadelphia 1977).

3 Morgan, P.G.M.; Turner-Warwick, M.: Pulmonary hemosiderosis and pulmonary hemorrhage. Br. J. Dis. Chest *75:* 225 (1981).

4 Virchow, R.: Die Krankhaften Geschwulste, p. 240 (August Hirshwald, Berlin 1864).

5 Ceelen, W.: Die Kreislaufstörungen der Lungen; in Henke, Lubarsch, Handbuch der speziellen pathologischen Anatomie und Histologie, vol. 3, p. 20 (Springer, Berlin 1931).

6 Soergel, K.H.; Sommers, S.C.: Idiopathic pulmonary hemosiderosis and related syndromes. Am. J. Med. *32:* 499 (1962).

7 Nickerson, M.J.: Idiopathic pulmonary hemosiderosis in a 5-month old infant. Clin. Pediat. *7:* 416 (1968).

8 Thaell, J.F.; Greipp, P.R.; Stubbs, S.E.; Siegal, G.P.: Idiopathic pulmonary hemosiderosis, two cases in a family. Mayo Clin. Proc. *53:* 113 (1978).

9 Beckerman, C.; Taussig, L.M.; Pinnas, L.: Familial idiopathic pulmonary hemosiderosis. Am. J. Dis. Child. *133:* 609 (1979).

10 Miller, T.; Tanaka, T.: Nuclear scan of pulmonary hemorrhage in idiopathic pulmonary hemosiderosis. Am. J. Roentge. *132:* 120 (1979).

11 Ewan, P.W.; Jones, H.A.; Rhodes, C.G.; Hughes, J.M.B.: Detection of intrapulmonary hemorrhage with carbon monoxide uptake. Application in Goodpasture's syndrome. New Engl. J. Med. *295:* 1391 (1976).

12 Donlan, C.J.; Srodes, C.H.; Duffy, F.D.: Idiopathic pulmonary hemosiderosis. Electron microscopic immunofluorescent and iron kinetic studies. Chest *68:* 577 (1975).

13 Allue, X.; Wise, M.B.; Baudry, P.H.: Pulmonary function studies in idiopathic pulmonary hemosiderosis in children. Am. Rev. resp. Dis. *107:* 410 (1973).

14 Irwin, R.S.; Cottrell, T.S.; Hsu, K.C.; Griswold, W.R.; Thomas, H.M.: Idiopathic pulmonary hemosiderosis: An electron microscopic and immunofluorescent study. Chest *65:* 41 (1974).

15 Yeager, H.; Powell, D.; Weinberg, R.M.; Bauer, H.; Bellanti, J.A.; Katz, S.: Idiopathic pulmonary hemosiderosis. Ultrastructural studies and response to azathioprine. Archs intern. Med. *136:* 1145 (1976).

16 Stafford, H.A.; Polmar, S.H.J.; Boat, T.F.: Immunologic studies in cow's milk-induced pulmonary hemosiderosis. Pediatrics, Springfield *11:* 898 (1977).

17 Soergel, K.H.; Sommers, S.C.: The alveolar epithelial lesion of idiopathic pulmonary hemosiderosis. Am. Rev. resp. Dis. *85:* 540 (1962).

18 Heiner, D.C.; Sears, J.W.; Kniker, W.T.: Multiple precipitins to cow's milk in chronic respiratory disease. A syndrome including poor growth, gastrointestinal symptoms, evidence of allergy, iron deficiency anemia and pulmonary hemosiderosis. Am. J. Dis. Child. *103:* 634 (1962).

19 Boat, T.F.; Polmar, S.H.; Whitman, V.; Kleinerman, J.I.; Stern, R.C.; Dershuk, C.F.: Hyper-reactivity to cow milk in young children with pulmonary hemosiderosis and cor pulmonale secondary to nasopharyngeal obstruction. J. Pediat. *87:* 22 (1975).

20 Lee, S.K.; Kniker, W.T.; Cook, C.D.; Heiner, D.C.: Cow's milk induced pulmonary disease in children; in Barness, Advances in pediatrics, vol. 25, pp. 39–57 (Year Book, Chicago 1978).

21 Bahna, S.I.; Heiner, D.C.: Allergies to milk (Grune & Stratton, New York 1980).

22 Goodpasture, E.W.: The significance of certain pulmonary lesions in relation to the etiology of influenza. Am. J. med. Sci. *158:* 863 (1919).

23 Lerner, R.A.; Glassock, R.J.; Dixon, F.J.: The role of anti-glomerular basement membrane antibody in the pathogenesis of human glomerulonephritis. J. exp. Med. *126:* 989 (1967).

24 Briggs, W.A.; Johnson, J.P.; Teichman, S.; Yeager, H.C.; Wilson, C.B.: Antiglomerular basement membrane antibody-mediated glomerulonephritis and Goodpasture's syndrome. Medicine *58:* 348 (1979).

25 Teague, C.A.; Doak, P.B.; Simpson, I.J.; Rainer, S.P.; Herdson, P.B.: Goodpasture's syndrome. An analysis of 29 cases. Kidney int. *13:* 492 (1978).

26 O'Connel, E.J.; Dower, J.C.; Burke, E.C.; Brown, A.L.; McCaughey, W.T.E.: Pulmonary hemorrhage-glomerulonephritis syndrome. Relationship to Goodpasture's syndrome with report of a case in a 9 year old girl. Am. J. Dis. Child. *108:* 302 (1964).

27 Ozsoylu, S.; Hicsonmez, G.; Berkel, I.; Say, B.; Tinaztepe, B.: Goodpasture's syndrome (Pulmonary hemosiderosis with nephritis). Clin. Pediat. *15:* 358 (1976).

28 Martini, A.; Binda, S.; Mariani, G.; Scotta, M.S.; Ruberto, G.: Goodpasture's syndrome in a child: Natural history and effect of treatment. Acta pediat. scand. *70:* 435 (1981).

29 Lewis, E.J.: Pulmonary hemorrhage and glomerulonephritis (Goodpasture's syndrome); in Edelmann, Pediatric kidney disease, vol. 2, pp. 736–745 (Little, Brown, Boston 1978).

30 Katzenstein, A.L.; Askin, F.B.: Surgical pathology of non-neoplastic lung disease, pp. 128–134 (Saunders, Philadelphia 1982).

31 Spargo, B.H.; Seymour, A.E.; Ordonez, N.G.: Renal biopsy pathology with diagnostic and therapeutic implications, pp. 191–204 (Wiley, New York 1980).

32 Agodoa, L.C.Y.; Striker, G.E.; George, C.R.P.; Glassock, R.; Quadracci, L.J.: The appearance of nonlinear deposits of immunoglobulins in Goodpasture's syndrome. Am. J. Med. *61:* 407 (1976).

33 Pasternack, A.; Tornroth, T.; Linder, E.: Evidence of both anti-GBM and immune complex mediated pathogenesis in the initial phase of Goodpasture's syndrome. Clin. Nephrol. *9:* 77 (1978).

34 Klassen, J.; Elwood, C.; Grossberg, A.L.; Milgrom, F.; Montes, M.; Sepulveda, M.; Andres, G.A.: Evolution of membranous nephropathy into anti-glomerular-basement-membrane glomerulonephritis. New Engl. J. Med. *290:* 1340 (1974).

35 Poskitt, T.R.: Immunologic and electron microscopic studies in Goodpasture's syndrome. Am. J. Med. *49:* 250 (1970).

36 Donald, K.J.; Edwards, R.L.; McEvoy, J.D.S.: Alveolar capillary basement membrane lesions in Goodpasture's syndrome and Idiopathic pulmonary hemosiderosis. Am. J. Med. *59:* 642 (1975).

37 McPhaull, J.J.; Dixon, F.J.: The presence of anti-glomerular basement membrane antibodies in peripheral blood. J. Immun. *103:* 1168 (1969).

38 Wilson, C.B.; Dixon, F.J.: Anti-glomerular basement membrane antibody induced glomerulonephritis. Kidney int. *3:* 74 (1973).

39 Unanue, E.R.; Dixon, F.J.: Experimental glomerulonephritis. Immunologic events and pathogenic mechanisms. Adv. Immunol. *6:* 1 (1967).

40 Wilson, C.B.; Smith, R.C.: Goodpasture's syndrome associated with influenza A₂ virus infection. Ann. intern. Med. *76:* 91 (1972).

41 Beirne, G.J.; Brennan, J.T.: Glomerulonephritis associated with hydrocarbon solvents. Mediated by anti-glomerular basement membrane antibody. Archs envir. Hlth *25:* 365 (1972).

42 Gossain, V.V.; Gerstein, A.R.; Janes, A.W.: Goodpasture's syndrome. A familial occurrence. Am. Rev. resp. Dis. *105:* 621 (1972).

43 Rees, A.J.; Peters, D.K.; Compston, D.A.S.; Batchelor, J.R.: Strong association between HLA-DRW₂ and antibody-mediated Goodpasture's syndrome. Lancet *i:* 966 (1978).

44 Yum, M.N.; Lampton, L.M.; Bloom, P.M.; Edwards, J.L.: Asymptomatic IgA nephropathy associated with pulmonary hemosiderosis. Am. J. Med. *64:* 1056 (1978).

45 Loughlin, G.M.; Taussig, L.M.; Murphy, S.A.; Strunk, R.C.; Kohnen, P.W.: Immune-complex-mediated glomerulonephritis and pulmonary hemorrhage simulating Goodpasture's syndrome. J. Pediat. *93:* 181 (1978).

46 Sternlieb, I.; Bennett, B.; Scheinberg, I.H.: *D*-Penicillamine induced Goodpasture's syndrome in Wilson's disease. Ann. intern. Med. *82:* 673 (1975).

47 Matthay, R.A.; Schwartz, M.I.; Petty, T.L.; Stanford, R.E.; Gupta, R.G.; Sahn, S.A.; Steigerwald, J.C.: Pulmonary manifestations of systemic lupus erythematosus. Review of twelve cases of acute lupus pneumonitis. Medicine *54:* 397 (1974).

48 Fayemi, A.O.: Pulmonary vascular disease in systemic lupus erythematosus. Am. J. clin. Path. *65:* 284 (1976).

49 Eagen, J.W.; Memoli, V.A.; Roberts, J.L.; Matthew, G.R.; Schwartz, M.M.; Lewis, E.J.: Pulmonary hemorrhage in systemic lupus erythematosus. Medicine *57:* 545 (1978).

50 Kuhn, C.: Systemic lupus erythematosus in a patient with ultrastructural lesions of the pulmonary capillaries previously reported in the review as due to idiopathic pulmonary hemosiderosis (Letter to the Editor). Am. Rev. resp. Dis. *106:* 931 (1982).

51 Rajami, K.B.; Ashbacher, L.V.; Kinney, T.R.: Pulmonary hemorrhage and systemic lupus erythematosus. J. Pediat. *93:* 810 (1978).

52 Elliot, M.L.; Kuhn, C.: Idiopathic pulmonary hemosiderosis. Ultrastructural abnormalities in the capillary walls. Am. Rev. resp. Dis. *102:* 895 (1970).

53 Leatherman, J.W.; Sibley, R.W.; Davies, S.F.: Diffuse intrapulmonary hemorrhage and glomerulonephritis unrelated to anti-glomerular basement membrane antibody. Am. J. Med. *72:* 401 (1982).

54 O'Donohue, W.J.: Idiopathic pulmonary hemosiderosis with manifestations of multiple connective tissue and immune disorders. Treatment with cyclophosphamide. Am. Res. resp. Dis. *109:* 473 (1974).

55 Schachter, E.N.; Finkelstein, F.O.; Bastl, C.; Walker-Smith, G.J.: Diagnostic problems in pulmonary-renal syndromes. Am. Rev. resp. Dis. *115:* 155 (1977).

56 Cunningham, R.; Hammond, D.: Pulmonary hemosiderosis associated with a collagen vascular syndrome. Am. J. Dis. Child. *102:* 643 (1961).

57 Perelman, R.; Nathanson, M.; Davis, F.; Hayem, F.; Gesnu, M.; Gondal, M.: Hémosiderose pulmonaire associée a une arthrite rheumatoid avec cellules LE. Sem. Hôp. Paris *55:* 1129 (1979).

58 Zollinger, H.U.; Heggelin, R.: Die idiopathische Lungen-Haemosiderose als pul-
    monale Form der Purpura Schönlein-Henoch. Schweiz. med. Wschr. *88:* 439 (1958).

59 Buchanan, G.R.; Moore, G.C.: Pulmonary hemosiderosis and immune throm-
    bocytopenia. Initial manifestations of collagen-vascular disease. J. Am. med. Ass. *246:*
    861 (1981).

60 Entieknap, J.B.: Lung biopsy in mitral stenosis. J. clin. Path. *6:* 84 (1953).

61 Heath, D.; Edwards, J.E.: The pathology of hypertensive pulmonary vascular disease.
    A description of six grades of structural changes in the pulmonary arteries with special
    reference to congenital cardiac septal defects. Circulation *18:* 533 (1958).

62 Utzon, F.; Brandrup, F.: Pulmonary arteriovenous fistulas in children. A review with
    special reference to the dispersed telangiectatic type, illustrated by report of a case.
    Acta pediat. scand. *62:* 422 (1973).

63 Wagenvoort, C.A.; Wagenvoort, N.: The pathology of pulmonary veno-occlusive dis-
    ease. Virchows Arch. Abt. A. Path. Anat. *364:* 69 (1974).

64 Corrin, B.; Liebow, A.A.; Friedman, P.J.: Lymphangiomyomatosis. A review. Am. J.
    Path. *79:* 348 (1975).

65 Wright, P.H.; Menzies, I.S.; Pounder, R.E.; Keeling, P.W.N.: Adult idiopathic pul-
    monary haemosiderosis and coeliac disease. Q. Jl. Med. *197:* 95 (1981).

66 Rieu, D.; Ariole, P.; Lesbros, D.; Emberger, J.M.; Jean, R.: Hemosidérose pul-
    monaire idiopathique et maladie cœliaque chez l'enfant. Une observation. Presse méd.
    12: 2931 (1983).

67 Ahmad, D.; Patterson, R.; Morgan, W.K.C.; Williams, T.; Zeiss, C.R.: Pulmonary
    haemorrhage and haemolytic anaemia due to trimellitic anhydride. Lancet *ii:* 328
    (1979).

68 Gonzales-Crussi, F.; Hull, M.T.; Grosfeld, J.L.: Idiopathic pulmonary hemosiderosis.
    Evidence of capillary basement membrane abnormality. Am. Rev. resp. Dis. *114:* 689
    (1976).

69 Valderrama, E.: Idiopathic pulmonary hemosiderosis (Abstract). Lab. Invest. *48:* 15P
    (1983).

70 Hyatt, R.W.; Adelstein, E.R.; Halazun, J.E.; Lukens, J.N.: Ultrastructure of the lung
    in idiopathic pulmonary hemosiderosis. Am. J. Med. *52:* 822 (1972).

71 Stejskal, J.; Pirani, C.L.; Okada, M.; Mandelanakis, N.; Pollak, V.E. Discontinuities
    (gaps) of the glomerular capillary wall and basement membrane in renal disease. Lab.
    Invest. *28:* 149 (1973).

72 Adamson, I.Y.R.; Bowden, D.H.: Derivation of type 1 epithelium from type 2 cells in
    the developing rat lung. Lab. Invest. *32:* 736 (1975).

73 Cutz, E.: Unpubl. observations.

74 Cutz, E.; Levison, H.; Cooper, D.H.: Ultrastructure of airways in children with
    asthma. Histopathology *2:* 407 (1978).

75 Lagunoff, D.: The role of mast cells in asthma. Expl. Lung Res. *4:* 121 (1983).

76 Bergofsky, E.H.: Humoral control of the pulmonary circulation. A. Rev. Physiol. *42:*
    221 (1980).

77 Ho, P.C.; Lewis, R.A.; Austen, K.F.; Orange, R.P.: Mediators of immediate hyper-
    sensitivity; in Gupta, Good, Cellular molecular and clinical aspects of allergic disor-
    ders, p. 179 (Plenum Press, New York 1979).

78 Richter, G.W.: The iron-loaded cell. The cytopathology of iron storage. A review.
    Am. J. Path. *91:* 363 (1978).

79 Finch, C.A.; Huebers, H.: Perspectives in iron metabolism. New Engl. J. Med. *306:* 1520 (1982).

80 Cohen, A.; Schwartz, E.: Decreasing iron stores during intensive chelation therapy. Ann. N.Y. Acad. Sci. *344:* 405 (1980).

81 Weibel, E.R.: How does lung structure affect gas exchange? Chest *83:* 657 (1983).

82 Hawkes, S.; Wang, J.L.: Extracellular matrix (Academic Press, New York 1982).

83 Gail, D.B.; Lenfant, C.J.M.: Cells of the lung. Biology and clinical implications. Am. Rev. resp. Dis. *127:* 366 (1983).

84 Battacharya, J.; Nanjo, S.; Staub, N.C.: Factors affecting lung microvascular injury. Ann. N.Y. Acad. Sci. *384:* 107–114 (1982).

Dr. E. Cutz, Department of Pathology, The Hospital for Sick Children, 555 University Avenue, Toronto, Ont. M5G 1X8 (Canada)

Perspect. pediatr. Pathol., vol. 11, pp. 82–96 (Karger, Basel 1987)

Pulmonary Lesions of Thalassemia Major

Benjamin H. Landing[a], *Rosario Nadorra*[a], *Carol B. Hyman*[b], *Jorge A. Ortega*[a]

[a]Departments of Pathology and Pediatrics, Children's Hospital of Los Angeles and University of Southern California School of Medicine, and
[b]Department of Pediatrics, Cedars-Sinai Medical Center, Los Angeles, Calif., USA

Introduction

To correlate pulmonary histopathologic alterations with pulmonary functional abnormalities in patients with thalassemia major [1–3], we analyzed the lung lesions in 14 patients dying of thalassemia major between 1958 and 1982.

Keens et al. [1], in studies of 12 patients with beta-thalassemia, found normal total lung capacity, but residual lung volume to be abnormally high in almost half. The single-breath nitrogen washout curve was also abnormal in half, despite normal closing volumes. The maximum expiratory flow rate at 60% total lung capacity was decreased in some, suggesting small airway disease. The most consistent finding was peripheral arterial hypoxemia, found in most of the patients.

Cooper et al. [2] studied 17 patients, with findings both similar to and different from those of Keens et al. [1]. Total lung capacity was frequently reduced, perhaps because of hepatomegaly. Reduced arterial oxygen saturation in most patients suggested ventilation-perfusion mismatching, but CO diffusion was usually above normal. Static and dynamic compliances were reduced, and lung recoil at total lung capacity was above normal. Upstream conductance was usually above normal. Cooper et al. [2] attributed the results to pulmonary fibrosis, despite lack of evidence of this lesion in a group of eight other patients studied post mortem. They thought the decreased lung compliance in their patients to be independent of the

Table I. Pulmonary lesions – patients with thalassemia

Patient No.	Year of death	Age years	Hemo-sideri-nophages	Respiratory epithelial and gland hemosiderin	Respiratory epithelial lipofuscin	Smooth muscle lipofuscin	Ferrugin-ation of connective tissues	Interstitial fibrosis
1	1967	9	+	0	0	0	0	0
2	1964	10	2+	−	+	+	0	2+
3	1958	12	+	+	0	−	+	−
4	1958	13	+	0	0	0	+	0
5	1972	14	+	+	2+	+	+	±
6	1963	15	3+	+	2+	−	+	+
7	1975	16	6+	+	+	±	4+	3+
8	1969	18	+	−	−	−	3+	+
9	1976	19	2+	+	−	−	±	2+
10	1973	23	3+	+	+	−	3+	2+
11	1982	25	2+	+	+	−	−	−
12	1984	26	+	+	−	−	−	−
13	1978	27	+	0	+	−	±	−
14	1980	28	3+	+	2+	±	2+	3+

±=Presence of lesion doubtful; +, 2+, 3+, 4+=degree of lesion mild, moderate, severe, very severe; −=lesion not present; 0=presence of lesion not evaluable in material available. Patients 12 and 14 are siblings.

reduced lung volume and peripheral air-space volume to be reduced in comparison with airway volume.

Wasi et al. [3] attributed low arterial oxygen levels in thalassemia to 'organized recanalized (pulmonary) thromboemboli', which had been found by Sonakul et al. [4] in 44% of patients dying with beta-thalassemia/ hemoglobin E disease in Thailand. These workers suggested that the thrombotic vascular lesions might have been the result of thrombocytosis following splenectomy [4].

Material and Methods

The material in the files of the Anatomic Pathology Division, Department of Laboratories, Children's Hospital of Los Angeles, from 14 patients who died of thalassemia major between 1958 and 1984 was reviewed and the findings were tabulated (table I, II). Paraffin sections of the available lung blocks were stained with hematoxylin and eosin,

Table II. Pulmonary lesions – patients with thalassemia

Patient No.	Year of death	Age years	'Sclerotic' vascular lesions	Recent/old thrombi	Emboli (marrow)	Angiectatic lesions (spider angiomas)	Chronic pneumonitis	Subpleural 'emphysema'	Acute edema	Cirrhosis of liver
1	1967	9	+	0	0	0	0	0	0	0
2	1964	10	–	–	–	–	3+	–	–	2+
3	1958	12	–	–	–	–	+	+	2+	0
4	1958	13	0	0	0	0	+	+	2+	0
5	1972	14	±	–	–	+	–	±	+	3+
6	1963	15	2+	–	–	+	2+	–	+	3+
7	1975	16	4+	0	–	+	+	2+	–	4+
8	1969	18	±	–	–	–	+	2+	–	4+
9	1976	19	+	+	–	±	+	2+	–	3+
10	1973	23	3+	+	+	+	0	+	0	2+
11	1982	25	–	+	–	+	–	–	–	3+
12	1984	26	–	–	–	+	–	–	–	2+
13	1978	27	±	–	–	+	–	0	–	2+
14	1980	28	3+	+	+	2+	±	+	–	3+

±=Presence of lesion doubtful; +, 2+ . . . 6+=degree of presence; –=lesion not present; 0=presence not evaluable in material available.

Gomori iron stain, Mallory trichrome stain, reticulum stain, and Scott sulfuric acid permanganate-aldehyde fuchsin stain.

The left lung of patient 12 was removed intact at autopsy and the left pulmonary artery was injected with a radioopaque silicone preparation (microfil MV-122, yellow, radioopaque; Canton Bio-Medical Products, Inc., Boulder, Colo.) at a pressure of 11 cm H_2O (8 mm Hg). The subpleural spider angiomata were demonstrated during the early phase of filling of the pulmonary vascular bed (fig. 15).

Pathologic Findings

Hemosiderinophages

All patients had pulmonary infiltrates of hemosiderinophages in varying degree, with a general tendency to increased severity with age and duration of disease. For example, hemosiderosis of 2+ or greater degree was present in 5 of 8 patients aged 16 or more and in only 2 of 6 patients below age 16. Hemosiderinophages occurred in alveolar spaces, but were

most abundant in the septa and perivascular sheaths (fig. 1). Since the infiltrates clearly increase the mass of lung tissue to be moved with each respiratory excursion, their presence presumably contributes to reduced pulmonary compliance.

Respiratory Epithelial and Glandular Hemosiderin

Hemosiderin was demonstrated in the respiratory epithelium or in the
cells of tracheal and bronchial glands of 10 of 11 evaluable patients (fig. 2),
with a tendency to increased frequency with age and duration of disease.
Although iron availability is considered to be a rate-limiting factor for the
growth of many bacteria, and the findings suggest that iron levels of airway
secretions and pulmonary tissues should be significantly elevated in patients of this type, acute bacterial infections of the respiratory tract or lung
are not important clinical aspects of thalassemia major, and acute
tracheitis, bronchitis, bronchiolitis and pneumonia were not components
of the terminal episode of any of the patients.

Epithelial and Smooth Muscle Lipofuscin

Lipofuscin in respiratory epithelial cells, respiratory glands, and
smooth muscle of blood vessels and airways was demonstrated by the sulfuric acid-permanganate-aldehyde fuchsin stain in 8 of the 11 evaluable patients. Lipofuscin was found more frequently in respiratory epithelial than
in smooth muscle cells (table I) (fig. 3), and all patients with smooth muscle deposits also had respiratory epithelial deposits. The increased lipofuscin formation results from iron catalysis of lipid peroxidation and perhaps
also from deficient vitamin E uptake secondary to the severe pancreatic atrophy and fat malabsorbtion regular in advanced thalassemia [5].

Ferrugination of Connective Tissues

Ferrugination of connective tissues, including alveolar septa, blood
vessels, and bronchial walls (fig. 4, 5), was demonstrated in 10 of 12 evaluable patients, increasing in severity with age and duration of disease. Ferrugination of connective tissue in the severely cirrhotic liver of patient 7
(fig. 6) indicates that the process affects connective tissues widely in the
body. Although the effect of this mineralizing process on the mechanical
properties of connective tissue matrices has apparently never been studied, we propose that a stiffening effect on both connective tissues and vascular walls could explain, at least in part, the reduced pulmonary compliance observed by Cooper et al. [2] in patients with thalassemia major.

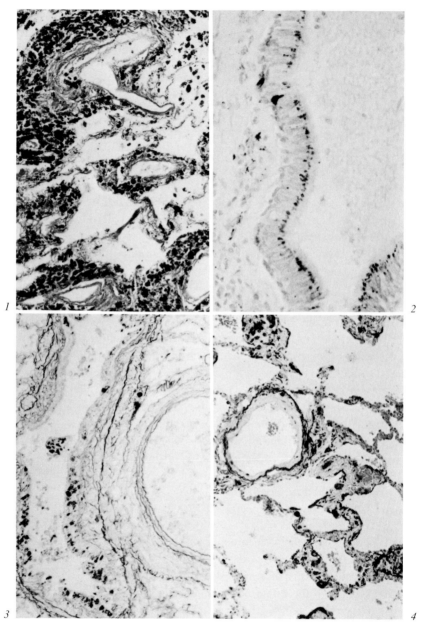

Fig. 1. Subpleural area of lung of patient 7, showing marked infiltration of interstitium and perivascular regions by hemosiderinophages, and multiple small dilated blood vessels. Reticulum stain. ×135.

Interstitial Fibrosis

Some degree of interstitial fibrosis of the lungs was observed in 8 of 12 evaluable patients, without a clear relationship to age and duration of disease. We did not establish the cause of this fibrosis, as the degree of interstitial fibrosis did not correlate with the degree of either vascular sclerosis or chronic pneumonitis. Certain enzymes involved in the post-translational modifications of procollagen are known to be iron catalyzed [6]. Our suspicion that ferrugination of connective tissue and vascular walls is a more important factor than pulmonary interstitial fibrosis in the reduced pulmonary compliance of patients with advanced thalassemia major requires confirmation.

Sclerotic Vascular Lesions and Thromboemboli

Sclerotic vascular lesions of several types were seen in 9 of 13 evaluable patients. Varying degrees of subendothelial hyaline thickening in small vessels appeared to result from ferrugination of vascular walls (fig. 1, 5, 6). Tortuous and thick-walled vessels contained thromboemboli in varying stages of organization (fig. 7, 8). These lesions recall those attributed by Sonakul et al. [4] in Hgb E/thalassemia to platelet thrombi. Since the majority of patients in this study were on a high-transfusion regimen [7], it is possible that some of the thrombi observed were actually emboli. Recent thrombi were identified in four patients and bone marrow emboli in two. Intimal proliferation (fig. 11) with multiple luminal channels (fig. 14) presumably resulting from organization and recanalization of thrombi.

Whether the various vascular lesions explain any of the pulmonary functional abnormalities reported in thalassemia by contributing to ventilation-perfusion imbalance or by affecting pulmonary compliance cannot be stated. However, collateral bronchial artery flow distal to the site(s) of pulmonary artery obstruction, the usual response to pulmonary artery occlusion, does not explain peripheral arterial oxygen unsaturation, the most common pulmonary functional abnormality in thalassemia major.

Fig. 2. Iron stain of small bronchus of patient 9, showing hemosiderin granules in apical region of bronchial epithelial cells. ×338.

Fig. 3. Small bronchus and adjacent pulmonary artery of patient 5, showing lipofuscin granules in bronchial epithelium, but no apparent lipofuscin in arterial smooth muscle. Sulfuric acid-permanganate aldehyde-fuchsin stain. ×135.

Fig. 4. Ferrugination of connective tissue and vascular walls in patient 1, demonstrated by overstaining with hematoxylin in HE stain. ×135.

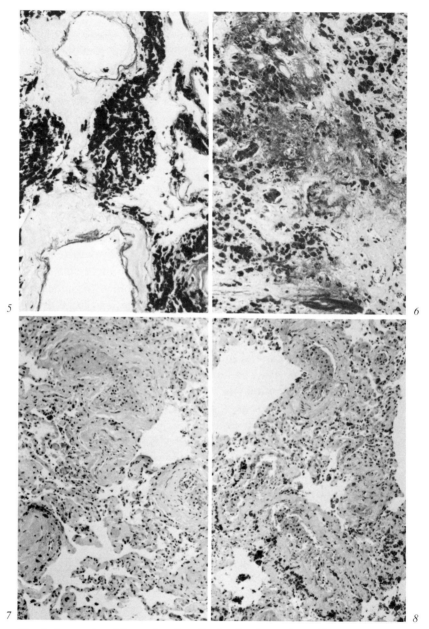

Fig. 5. Iron stain of lung of patient 7, showing heavy interstitial infiltration by hemosiderinophages, ferrugination of subendothelial connective tissue of blood vessels, and hyaline thickening of vessel walls seen in association with vascular ferrugination. ×135.

Angiectatic Lesions Consistent with 'Spider' Arteriovenous Fistulae

Vascular dilatations consistent with spider angiomas of the lung were found in 9 of the 12 evaluable patients (fig. 12–14); all 9 were aged 14 years or older (table II). Some vessels also showed the hyaline intimal thickening associated with ferrugination of vascular walls (fig. 12). Pulmonary arteriovenous fistulas of spider-angioma type accompany various diseases producing cirrhosis of the liver [8–13] and are considered to be the explanation of the peripheral arterial oxygen unsaturation, cyanosis and digital clubbing frequently seen in cirrhotic patients. Hepatic cirrhosis was present in all 11 evaluable patients in this series (table II). Subpleural spider angiomata with arteriovenous shunting were demonstrated by injection of the left pulmonary artery of patient 12 (fig. 15). The findings are comparable to those of other workers using similar injection methods on specimens from patients with other types of hepatic cirrhosis [8, 9, 12]. We propose that appropriate physiologic studies during life [13] will further demonstrate that such arteriovenous shunts explain the peripheral arterial oxygen unsaturation of patients with thalassemia major [1–3].

Chronic Pneumonitis

Nine of 12 evaluable patients had chronic pneumonitis with interstitial lymphoid infiltration, macrophage exudation into alveolar lumens, or both, although to a significant degree in only 2 (fig. 16). None had viral inclusions.

Subpleural Emphysema

Enlarged subpleural air spaces were present in 8 of the 12 evaluable patients in the series (fig. 17). Their occurrence in patients dying before the early 1970s might reflect overventilation due to anemia, but this mechanism does not explain the occurrence in patients dying more recently, as

---

Fig. 6. Ferrugination of connective tissue of severely cirrhotic liver of same patient as in figure 5, to demonstrate the widespread ferrugination of connective tissue seen in patients with thalassemia who have advanced hemosiderosis. Iron stain. ×135.

Fig. 7. Subpleural region of lung of patient 12 showing variable interstitial and alveolar septal fibrosis, perivascular fibrosis, and thick-walled tortuous vessels consistent with healing thromboemboli. HE. ×135.

Fig. 8. Lung of same patient as in figure 7, showing organizing stages of endovascular material consistent with thromboemboli, as well as a degree of perivascular and interstitial fibrosis. HE. ×135.

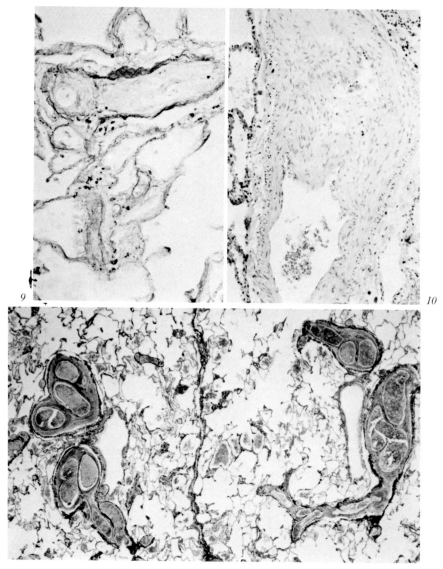

Fig. 9. Vessel in lung of patient 10, showing narrowing and partial obliteration of lumen, consistent with a late stage of organization of thrombus. Sulfuric acid-permanganate aldehyde-fuchsin stain. ×135.

Fig. 10. Vessel in lung of same patient as in figure 9, showing changes consistent with late stage of organization of thrombus. HE. ×135.

Fig. 11. Multichanneled vessels typical of organized thrombi in lung of patient 10. Reticulum stain. ×34.

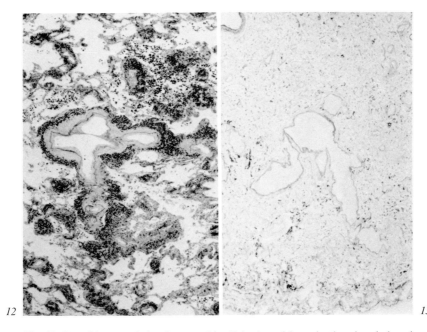

12   13

Fig. 12. Branching vessel showing mural hyalinization of ferrugination, in subpleural region of lung of patient 7. The shape of the vessel is consistent with that of the central vessel in a spider angioma. HE. ×34.

Fig. 13. Branching vessel consistent with subpleural spider angioma in patient 9. Aldehyde fuchsin stain. ×34.

they received frequent transfusions to maintain hemoglobin concentrations [7]. Possible explanations include: (a) reduced alpha-1-antitrypsin or other antiprotease production as the result of hepatic cirrhosis; (b) release of pancreatic elastase, trypsin, or other proteases as the result of pancreatic involvement in thalassemia; (c) increased leukocyte protease activity, secondary to postsplenectomy leukocytosis, possibly enhanced by reduced hepatic antiprotease production [15–18]; (d) the effect of increased tissue iron and reduced vitamin E on inactivation of antiproteases in the lung [19].

Pulmonary Edema
Four patients, 3 of whom died before high-transfusion therapy regimens were introduced (table II), had pulmonary edema, probably as the result of heart failure due to anemia.

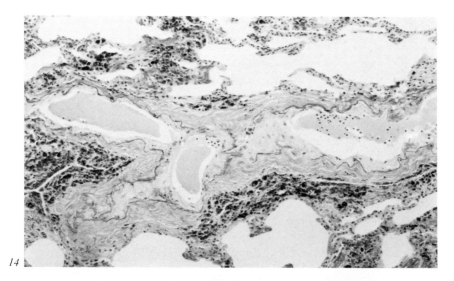

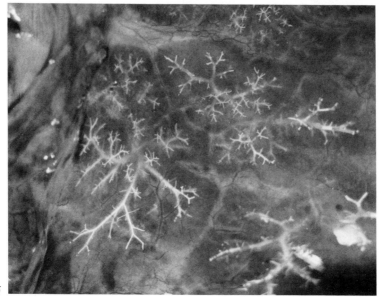

Fig. 14. Vessel consistent with 'stem vessel' of spider angioma, in subpleural region of lung of patient 7. The vessel also shows ferrugination of mural components, and the associated variable hyaline intimal thickening. HE. ×135.

Fig. 15. Subpleural spider angiomata (arterio-venous shunts) in subpleural tissue of lower lobe of patient 12, showing the filling of these shunts by material injected into the main pulmonary artery before the general parenchymal vascular bed is injected. ×1.

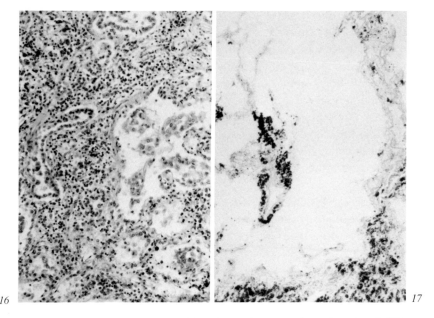

16   17

Fig. 16. Chronic interstitial pneumonitis with alveolar macrophages in patient 2. HE. ×135.

Fig. 17. Elongated and enlarged subpleural airspace in patient 7 showing remnants of alveolar septa projecting into lumen. The figure also shows interstitial and pleural infiltration by hemosiderinophages. Reticulum stain. ×135.

Other Lesions

Abnormally thin arterial walls were seen in several patients, but were not specifically tabulated (fig. 3, 15). Will [20] reported reduction in pulmonary arterial muscle thickness in the condition of 'oxidant stress'. Increased free radical production in patients with thalassemia major, secondary to iron catalysis of lipid peroxidation, and vitamin E deficiency, secondary to hyperconsumption or deficient absorbtion of vitamin E [5], may well produce the same effect as 'oxidant stress'. The amount of smooth muscle in peripheral airways seemed abnormally scanty in several of the patients in this study, but we did not validate the observation morphometrically.

Conclusion

Our review of the pulmonary lesions in 14 patients dying of thalassemia major demonstrated pulmonary hemosiderinophages, respiratory epithelial and glandular hemosiderosis, respiratory epithelial and smooth muscle lipofuscin accumulation, ferrugination of connective tissues of pulmonary interstitium, alveolar septal and blood vessels and pulmonary interstitial fibrosis. The pulmonary hemosiderinophage infiltration, ferrugination of connective tissues and interstitial fibrosis appears to explain the reduced pulmonary compliance reported in some patients with thalassemia major.

Vascular lesions included intimal thickening associated with mural ferrugination, organized thrombi, and spider angiomas like those reported in patients with other types of hepatic cirrhosis. Spider angiomas, by producing pulmonary arteriovenous shunting, appear to explain peripheral arterial oxygen unsaturation, the most commonly reported 'pulmonary' functional abnormality in patients with thalassemia major.

Chronic pneumonitis, acute pulmonary edema, and mild subpleural air-space emphysema were also found in some of the patients. Possible roles of deficient hepatic antiprotease production, of excessive pancreatic protease release or excessive leukocyte protease release in the lungs, and of inhibition of antiproteases in the pathogenesis of this emphysema are suggested.

The pulmonary lesions of thalassemia major differ in several ways from those of sickle cell anemia or hemoglobin SC disease, the most common of the structural hemoglobinopathies. Pulmonary artery thromboemboli are found in both sickling disorders and thalassemia major, and appear to be the most important pulmonary lesion in the sickle hemoglobinopathies, with frequent production of cor pulmonale, whereas pulmonary hemosiderinophage infiltration, ferrugination of connective tissues and vessels, and spider angiomata are more important pulmonary lesions in thalassemia major.

Acknowledgements

We are indebted to Mrs. Peggy Earhart for secretarial assistance, and to Miss Jacqueline Sedler for help in the pulmonary artery injection procedure.

References

1   Keens, T.G.; O'Neal, M.W.; Ortega, J.A.; Hyman, C.B.; Platzker, A.C.G.: Pulmonary function abnormalities in thalassemia patients on a hypertransfusion program. Pediatrics, Springfield 65: 1013–1017 (1980).

2   Cooper, D.M.; Mansell, A.L.; Weiner, M.A.; Berdon, W.E.; Chetty-Baktavisiam, A.; Reid, L.; Mellins, R.B.: Low lung capacity and hypoxemia in children with thalassemia major. Am. Rev. resp. Dis. 121: 639–646 (1980).

3   Wasi, P.; Fucharoen, S.; Youngchaiyud, P.; Sonakul, D.: Hypoxemia in thalassemia. Birth Defects, Orig. Article Ser. 18: 213–217 (1982).

4   Sonakul, D.; Pacharee, P.; Laohapand, T.; Fucharoen, S.; Wasi, P.: Pulmonary artery obstruction in thalassemia. Southeast Asian J. trop. Med. Publ. Hlth 11: 516–523 (1980).

5   Hyman, C.B.; Landing, B.H.; Alfin-Slater, R.; Kozak, L.; Weitzman, J.; Ortega, J.A.: dl-α-Tocopherol, iron, and lipofuscin in thalassemia. Third conference on Cooley's anemia. N.Y. Acad. Sci. 232: 211–220 (1974).

6   Iancu, T.C.; Landing, B.H.; Neustein, H.B.: Pathogenetic mechanisms in hepatic cirrhosis of thalassemia major. Light and electron microscopic studies. Pathol. A. 12: 171–200 (1977).

7   Hyman, C.B.; Ortega, J.A.; Costin, G.; Landing, B.H.; Lazerson, J.; Leimbrock, S.; Lurie, P.: Management of thalassemia in Los Angeles. Birth Defects, Orig. Article Ser. 7: 43–52 (1976).

8   Berthelot, P.; Walker, J.G.; Sherlock, S.; Reid, L.: Arterial changes in the lungs in cirrhosis of the liver-lung spider nevi. New Engl. J. Med. 274: 291–298 (1966).

9   Rydell, R.; Hoffbauer, F.W.: Multiple pulmonary arteriovenous fistulas in juvenile cirrhosis. Am. J. Med. 21: 450–460 (1956).

10   Bashour, F.A.; Cochran, P.: Alveolar-arterial oxygen tension gradients in cirrhosis of the liver. Further evidence of existing pulmonary arteriovenous shunting. Am. Heart J. 71: 734–740 (1966).

11   Keren, G.; Boichis, H.; Zwas, T.S.; Frand, M.: Pulmonary arterio-venous fistulae in hepatic cirrhosis. Archs Dis. Childh. 58: 302–304 (1983).

12   Kravath, R.E.; Scarpelli, E.M.; Bernstein, J.: Hepatogenic cyanosis. Arteriovenous shunts in chronic active hepatitis. J. Pediat. 78: 238–245 (1971).

13   Genovesi, M.G.; Tierney, D.F.; Toplin, G.V.; Eisenberg, H.: An intravenous radionucleide method to evaluate hypoxemia caused by abnormal alveolar vessels. Limitation of conventional techniques. Am. Rev. resp. Dis. 114: 59–65 (1976).

14   Geokas, M.; Rinderknecht, H.; Swanson, V.; Haverback, B.: The role of elastase in acute hemorrhagic pancreatitis in man. Clin. Res. 16: 151 (1968).

15   Janoff, A.: Proteases and lung injury. A state-of-the-art minireview. Chest 5: suppl., lung defense, injury and repair, pp. 545–585 (1983).

16   Hoidal, J.R.; Niewoehner, D.E.: The role of tissue repair and leucocytes in the pathogenesis of emphysema. Chest 5: suppl., lung defense, injury and repair, pp. 585–605 (1983).

17   Lonky, S.A.; McCarren, J.: Neutrophile enzymes in the lung. Regulation of neutrophile elastase. Am. Rev. resp. Dis. 127: 510–515 (1983).

18   Sandhaus, R.A.; McCarthy, K.M.; Masson, R.A.; Henson, P.M.: Elastolytic proteases of the human macrophage. Chest 5: suppl., lung defense, injury and repair, pp. 605–625 (1983).

19 Janoff, A.; Carp, H.; Laurent, P.; Roju, L.: The role of oxidative processes in emphysema. Am. Rev. resp. Dis. *127:* 531–538 (1983).

20 Will, J.A.: Neuroendocrine and metabolic factors affecting the circulation and airways of the lung. The Endocrine Lung in Health and Disease – An International Conf., Washington 1982.

21 Openheimer, E.H.; Esterly, J.R.: Pulmonary changes in sickle cell disease. Am. Rev. resp. Dis. *103:* 858–859 (1971).

22 Bomberg, P.A.: Pulmonary aspects of sickle cell disease. Archs intern. Med. *133:* 652–657 (1974).

23 Collins, F.S.; Orringer, E.P.: Pulmonary hypertension and cor pulmonale in the sickle hemoglobinopathies. Am. J. Med. *73:* 814–821 (1982).

B.H. Landing, MD, Anatomic Pathology Division,
Children's Hospital of Los Angeles,
4650 Sunset Boulevard, Los Angeles, CA 90027 (USA)

Perspect. pediatr. Pathol., vol. 11, pp. 97–123 (Karger, Basel 1987)

Mucosal Biopsy of the Esophagus in Children

Beverly Barrett Dahms, Fred C. Rothstein

Departments of Pathology and Pediatrics, Case Western Reserve University School of Medicine and Rainbow Babies and Children's Hospital, Cleveland, Ohio, USA

The development of small flexible endoscopes has so increased the number of endoscopic procedures and small mucosal biopsies in children that esophageal biopsies have become commonplace in our surgical pathology laboratory. Most esophageal mucosal biopsies are obtained from children undergoing evaluation for gastroesophageal reflux, infectious esophagitis, and the esophageal disorders arising in children with cancer.

Methods of Biopsy

Esophageal biopsies from children undergoing endoscopy for evaluation of esophageal disease are usually taken from two levels: one approximately 2–3 cm above the lower esophageal sphincter (LES) and another several centimeters higher, avoiding the distal esophagus within 2 cm of the lower esophageal sphincter because of its normal background of inflammatory cells and variation in site of the squamocolumnar junction. Typically, several pieces of tissue from each level are placed in the same container of fixative identified as to its location relative to the LES. Many esophageal biopsies in children obtained under direct visualization with grasp forceps are quite small, sometimes no more than fragments, and often consist only of the squamous epithelial layer. Usually, the biopsies are placed directly into fixative without orientation; the histotechnologist attempts orientation during embedding. Larger biopsies may be mounted and oriented on nylon mesh or filter paper. Most biopsies are obtained by grasp forceps which permits sampling multiple areas in a short period of time. The grasp forceps is passed through the endoscope. Suction biopsies are larger, deeper, and easier to orient prior to fixation but are not often performed in infants and small children since localization of the site requires direct visualization and passage of a suction biopsy capsule next to the endoscope. Discomfort to the child is increased, and procedure time is increased over that of the grasp biopsy technique.

The tissue may be fixed in any standard fixative: formalin, Zenker's and Bouin's solutions. Hematoxylin and eosin stained slides are usually adequate for evaluation, recognizing the variable appearance of eosinophils with different fixatives and different brands and dye lots of eosin. A 'ribbon' of serial sections is prepared from each paraffin block, sampling well into the center of the tissue. Our routine of examining five glass slides, each containing a ribbon of sections from each block, overcomes many of the shortcomings of the small size and random orientation of grasp biopsies.

Normal Esophageal Mucosa

Normal esophageal mucosa [1–3] has a nonkeratinized stratified squamous epithelium, a lamina propria of loose connective tissue, and a muscularis mucosa. The thin squamous epithelium of the neonate rapidly develops the mature thickness and appearance (fig. 1). The basal or proliferative layers of epithelium with its polyhedral cells, large round nuclei and reduced cytoplasmic glycogen appears darker and more basophilic than the superficial layers. The basal layers normally constitute no more than 15–20% of total epithelial thickness [4, 5]. The superficial layers of epithelium have flattened cells with thin, compact nuclei and pale glycogen-filled cytoplasm. In disorders such as esophagitis accompanied by more rapid shedding of superficial cells than normal, the basal layer becomes noticeably deeper, often constituting 50% or more of epithelial thickness. Normally, papillae of lamina propria project superficially at regular intervals never extending into the epithelium more than half of its total thickness. If sectioned tangentially, these papillae may appear as islands of connective tissue with blood vessels within the epithelium. Papillary elongation occurs regularly in esophagitis.

Familiarity with the normal esophagogastric squamocolumnar junction is essential for the interpretation of biopsies from the distal esophagus. The transition between squamous and columnar mucosa is usually

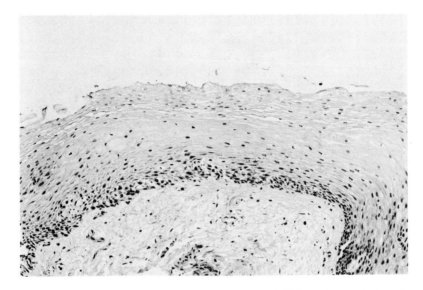

Fig. 1. Normal esophageal mucosa. Most of the epithelial thickness is occupied by cells with an elongate, compressed nucleus and abundant cytoplasm. Basal cells have larger, rounder nuclei and comparatively less cytoplasm than more superficial cells. The basal cell layer occupies less than 20% of total epithelial thickness. Occasional lymphocytes in lamina propria and epithelium are normal. HE. ×170.

sharp and circumferential, but a zigzag transition zone may extend over one or two centimeters. Biopsy of an irregular transition zone can lead to a jumble of squamous and gastric cardiac mucosae. The normal esophageal lamina propria contains occasional gastric cardiac-type mucous glands near the gastroesophageal junction; their presence at the junction does not constitute metaplasia. The lamina propria and even the squamous epithelium near the squamocolumnar junction normally contain occasional lymphocytes, but not neutrophils, eosinophils or plasma cells.

Gastroesophageal Reflux and Esophagitis

During the first few months of life, gastroesophageal reflux (GER) [6–9] commonly occurs because of immature esophageal function presenting as effortless regurgitation often controlled with postural therapy and thickened feedings. Specific medications to improve lower esophageal sphincter tone are occasionally necessary but most infants develop normal esophageal function during the first year of life, after which GER does not present a problem.

Persistent GER may lead to esophagitis and numerous complications throughout childhood, e.g. failure to thrive (from excessive caloric losses secondary to chronic vomiting) and recurrent respiratory disorders (asthma, aspiration pneumonitis, chronic bronchitis) [10, 11]. Common symptoms of esophagitis occurring after infancy include abdominal pain, heartburn and vomiting. Although children may not describe heartburn, they may complain of chest or abdominal pain, refuse to eat, or become irritable with meals, have foul breath in the morning, increased eructation, and episodes of hiccuping.

Clinical evaluation of GER and esophagitis includes barium esophagram with examination for reflux, even though it identifies GER in only 50% of symptomatic children. An upper GI series is also done to rule out gastric outlet obstruction. Esophageal pH monitoring is more sensitive than radiographic studies to document reflux. Endoscopy with biopsy is the most sensitive diagnostic procedure of all, and the only means of detecting esophagitis (as opposed to reflux). Erythema, friability, granularity and ulceration are not observed endoscopically in up to 30% of children who have symptomatic and histologic evidence of esophagitis [12]. Since the histology provides a mainstay in the diagnosis of reflux esophagitis, a biopsy is indicated in children with symptoms severe enough to warrant endoscopy. Most infants and children who develop GER are otherwise healthy, but certain groups are predisposed, including children with mental retardation [6], cystic fibrosis [13, 14], and esophageal atresia and tracheoesophageal fistula [15]. Even after successful surgical repair of esophageal atresia in the neonatal period, children with congenital esophageal atresia are prone to later esophageal problems, including GER.

Histology of Gastroesophageal Reflux

Histologic features of reflux esophagitis in children [12, 16] are similar to those in adults [2–5, 17, 18]. In 100 sequential pediatric biopsies performed at our hospital for symptomatic GER during 1983, symptomatic patients usually showed at least two of the salient features: (1) intraepithelial inflammation, primarily lymphocytic; (2) intraepithelial eosinophils [19]; (3) hyperplasia of the epithelial basal layer (>25% total thickness) [5]; (4) nuclear enlargement and hyperchromicity and edema within the basal layer; (5) telangiectasia [20], and (6) increased (>50%) penetration

Table I. Histologic findings in 100 consecutive esophageal biopsies in symptomatic children with gastroesophageal reflux

	Number
1 Intraepithelial lymphocytes or squiggle cells	95
2 Intraepithelial eosinophils	40
3 Basal cell hyperplasia >30%[1]	32
4 Basal cell nuclear changes, spongiosis	67
5 Telangiectasia	63
6 Papillary elongation >50% epithelial thickness[1]	37

[1] Could not be evaluated in many patients because of random orientation in superficial grasp biopsies.

of lamina propria papillae toward the epithelial surface [5] as superficial cell layers are lost (table I). Only the most severe cases and those in whom suction biopsies are taken have all of these features. Suction biopsies can be oriented during embedding, allowing accurate evaluation of basal layer thickness and papillary height. In small fragmented grasp biopsies, which usually consist of strips of suboptimally oriented squamous epithelium, the thickness of the basal layer and papillary height cannot be accurately measured but the other features remain identifiable. Milder lesions usually have a combination of basal layer changes and intraepithelial inflammation. To be significant, inflammation must be intraepithelial; the normal scattered lymphocytes in esophageal lamina propria have no diagnostic import nor does occasional intraepithelial mononuclear cells without one of the other features.

Histologic diagnosis of GER in the adult has been based on indication of irritation and rapid epithelial turnover, i.e. basal cell hyperplasia and increased papillary height in the absence of inflammation [4]. In our studies, most children with symptomatic GER have intraepithelial inflammation, in some children as the only histologic abnormality, although most children have more than one feature.

The mildest diagnostic alterations in GER usually include intraepithelial inflammation plus basal layer changes (fig. 2). As the rate of superficial epithelial cell shedding increases with acid reflux, the actively proliferating basal layer forms more than the expected normal 20% of epithe-

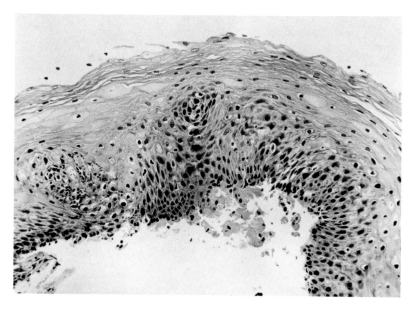

Fig. 2. Mild reflux esophagitis. This esophageal grasp biopsy consists only of a strip of randomly oriented stratified squamous epithelium, yet shows intraepithelial inflammatory cells and enlargement and hyperchromatism of basal cell nuclei. HE. ×200.

lial thickness. Focal basal cells may have nuclear enlargement and hyperchromatism. Intraepithelial inflammation usually consists of lymphocytes, 'squiggle cells', and eosinophils, less commonly neutrophils, unless ulceration has supervened. 'Squiggle cells' are distorted inflammatory cells of indeterminate type, probably lymphocytes or degranulated neutrophils, possibly crushed during grasp biopsy.

Intraepithelial eosinophils are a valuable and perhaps specific diagnostic criterion of reflux esophagitis. In the widely quoted paper of Winter et al. [19] sequential pH probe study and esophageal biopsy in a group of children showed that esophageal intraepithelial eosinophils were a highly specific indicator of acid reflux. Because of their high visibility, eosinophils may be identified with certainty even on the smallest and most poorly oriented specimens. The incidence of eosinophils among the inflammatory cells varies widely. They may be the only intraepithelial inflammatory cells or they may be admixed with lymphocytes and squiggle cells. Although intraepithelial eosinophils correlate with acid reflux, their absence does

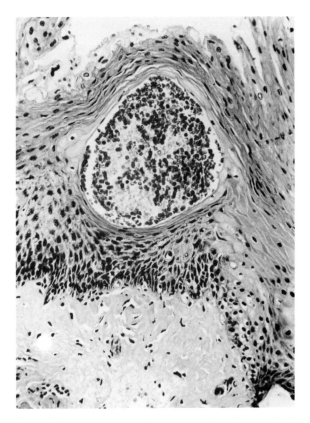

Fig. 3. Telangiectasia in the lamina propria in reflux esophagitis. When lamina propria papillae bearing these capillaries are tangentially sectioned, as in this photograph, the dilated vessel may appear isolated within the epithelium. HE. ×200.

not preclude reflux esophagitis. In Winter's study and in ours [19], 40–50% of the children with reflux had intraepithelial eosinophils in an esophageal mucosal biopsy. The reason for the variation in infiltrate by eosinophils remains unclear. Some cases of advanced reflux esophagitis with ulceration and stricture formation had no eosinophils. The number of eosinophils does not correlate well with severity of symptoms, the treatment, or the other histologic features.

Telangiectasia occurs nonspecifically with esophagitis [20], within papilla of lamina propria, and may signal subtle examples of GER (fig. 3). Tangential sections of the papillae bearing telangiectatic vessels may re-

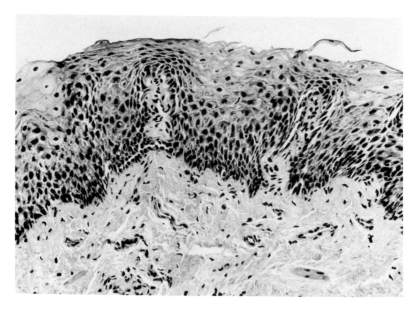

Fig. 4. Moderate reflux esophagitis. This well oriented suction biopsy shows basal layer hyperplasia, increase in papillary height to more than 50% of epithelial thickness, and intraepithelial inflammatory cells. HE. ×200.

veal thin-walled vessels as blood islands within the stratified squamous epithelium. They serve as a diagnostic clue in borderline cases and in randomly oriented grasp biopsy specimens.

With moderately advanced reflux esophagitis, all morphologic features become more prominent (fig. 4). As viewed in optimally oriented sections, papillae of lamina propria have increased height, often extending to more than 50% of epithelial thickness. In some cases of esophagitis, these papillae are separated from the surface by only a few epithelial cells. Increased papillary height and telangiectasia account for the erythema apparent by endoscopy.

With severe GER (fig. 5, 6) the increased rate of surface shedding and basal cell proliferation results in the basal layer occupying nearly 100% of epithelial thickness. Basal cell spongiosus accounts for the mucosal edema and friability identified endoscopically. Ulceration with GER (fig. 7) has been observed occasionally at endoscopy, but since histology of the ulcer bed shows only nonspecific necrosis and inflammation, biopsy of the surrounding epithelium provides more revealing information.

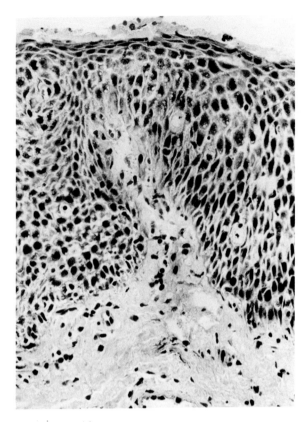

Fig. 5. Severe reflux esophagitis. Hyperplastic basal cell layer occupies nearly the entire epithelial thickness which also has spongiosis and intraepithelial inflammatory cells. Papillary height is increased. HE. ×300.

We do not interpret GER in an esophageal biopsy unless it contains two or more of the characteristic histologic features (table I). Since GER affects the lower one-third of the esophagus, at least one biopsy should be obtained 2 or 3 cm proximal to the LES. Since the mucosa contains occasional inflammatory cells near the squamocolumnar junction, biopsy at two levels is preferred. Most of our patients with GER showed histologic changes equally severe in both low (2–3 cm above the LES) and high (4–5 cm above the LES) biopsy specimens. In the presence of equivocal findings, we choose to err on the side of normality, since a diagnosis of GER leads to an initiation or continuation of medication, or, the consideration of antireflux surgery.

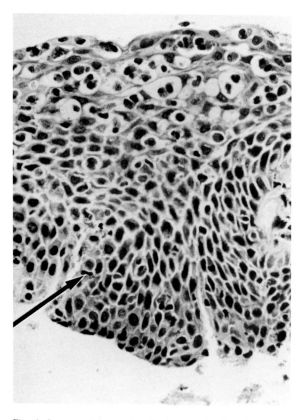

Fig. 6. Severe reflux esophagitis in a randomly oriented strip of epithelium reveals marked abundant, spongiosis, intraepithelial eosinophils near the surface and a squiggle cell (arrow). HE. ×480.

Differential Diagnosis of Gastroesophageal Reflux

The limited histopathologic differential diagnosis of reflux esophagitis includes occasional cases of infectious esophagitis in otherwise healthy nonimmunosuppressed children. With herpetic esophagitis (see below), the involvement may not be in continuity with the GE junction, as it is in reflux. An infiltrate of eosinophils in the lamina propria and epithelium of the esophagus may rarely [18] accompany eosinophilic gastroenteritis which, however, usually manifests more distally in the gastrointestinal tract, particularly in the gastric antrum and pylorus [21–24].

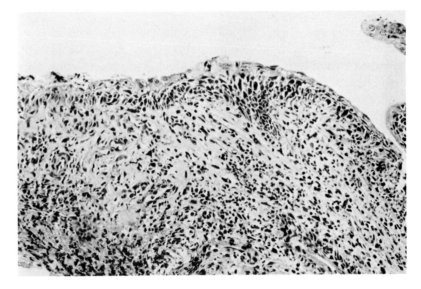

Fig. 7. Severe reflux esophagitis with ulceration at left. The intact epithelium (right) is atrophic. Lamina propria is densely inflamed. HE. ×200.

Ingestion of caustic substances such as alkaline drain cleaner (sodium hydroxide, ammonium hydroxide) and acids (sulfuric, hydrochloric) induces acute esophagitis and, after healing, may lead to esophageal dysfunction and gastroesophageal reflux. Although unusual, Crohn's disease may rarely involve the esophagus [25–27]. Apthous ulcerations separated from each other by normal appearing tissue may suggest Crohn's disease. Dermatologic conditions which may affect the esophagus include pemphigus, bullous pemphigoid and epidermolysis bullosa. Immunosuppressed or severely debilitated patients are more likely to have infectious esophagitis than GER.

Sequelae of Gastroesophageal Reflux

Severe GER may cause linear or irregular ulcers, nearly always in the distal one-third of the esophagus, resulting in chronic blood loss or even acute hemorrhage. Pseudopolyps or fibrotic strictures may follow prolonged GER with severe ulceration. Of all the sequelae of GER, Barrett's esophagus has incited the most current interest.

Barrett's Esophagus

Barrett's esophagus, metaplastic columnar epithelium in the distal esophagus resulting from chronic gastroesophageal reflux [28–30], has been recognized for three decades in adults, but until recently columnar epithelium in the esophagus of a child has been regarded as a congenital malformation. In his original description, Barrett [31] called it a congenitally short esophagus with partial intrathoracic stomach. Evidence for the acquired nature of Barrett's esophagus derived from development and progression of columnar epithelial metaplasia in adults with reflux [30] and experimentally in animals [32, 33].

In our studies of esophageal biopsies from 205 children and adolescents aged 8 months to 19 years, performed over a 6-year period (1978–1983) for evaluation of GER [34, 35], 17 (8.3%) had Barrett's esophagus. The occurrence of Barrett's esophagus has not been predicted from clinical history, but in about half of the patients the columnar epithelium was predicted by the endoscopic appearance of a salmon-pink mucosa contrasting with the surrounding erythematous, friable inflamed mucosa. In the other half, the columnar area could not be identified endoscopically. In all cases, the columnar epithelium was located in the distal one-third of the esophagus in continuity with the gastroesophageal junction.

Barrett's esophagus may have three types of columnar-lined mucosa [36]: (1) gastric fundic mucosa (fig. 8) complete with coiled glands containing parietal and chief cells; (2) junctional mucosa (fig. 9) resembling gastric cardia, and (3) specialized columnar mucosa (fig. 10, 11) resembling small intestine with a villiform surface and goblet cells. The specialized columnar mucosa superficially resembles the intestinal metaplasia found in adults with atrophic gastritis, except that the glands are cardiac mucous type rather than intestinal glands. Usually, the three types of Barrett mucosa are distinct from one another, but some biopsies have features of two types, e.g. fundic and cardiac glands may be admixed or gastric mucosa may contain occasional goblet cells.

The most commonly encountered mucosa was gastric fundic, present in 13 of 17 children in our cases of Barrett's esophagus, followed by junctional epithelium in 9 of the 17. Two of the older teenage patients had specialized columnar epithelium. In patients with multiple biopsies taken from different levels at the same endoscopy session, 1 patient had all three types of Barrett's epithelium and 3 patients had two types of epithelium. The distribution of the different types of Barrett's epithelium in relation to the LES conformed to the distribution regularly found in adults, i.e. gas-

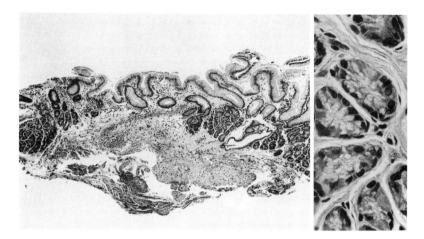

Fig. 8. Barrett's esophagus, gastric fundic type. The surface epithelium is tall columnar and the glands are coiled, with distinct parietal and chief cells (inset, right). This mucosa shows patchy glandular atrophy and diffuse inflammation. HE. ×110. Inset: ×600.

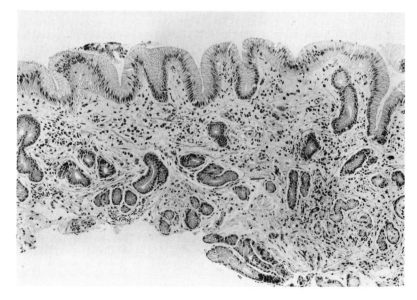

Fig. 9. Barrett's esophagus, gastric cardiac type. Surface epithelium is similar to gastric fundic type (fig. 8), but glands here are of gastric cardiac (mucous) type. HE. ×100.

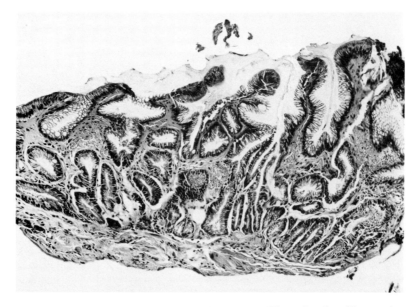

Fig. 10. Barrett's esophagus, specialized columnar type. The surface has villous projections similar to those in small intestine. Few goblet cells in the surface epithelium. HE. ×115.

tric fundic is most distal (nearest the LES), specialized columnar is most proximal, and junctional lies between.

The biopsy site must be established before making a diagnosis of Barrett's esophagus. Of the three histologic types of Barrett's epithelium, only the specialized columnar type is distinctive. Gastric fundic and junctional types must be distinguished from normal gastric mucosa, particularly near the squamocolumnar junction. Most cases have sufficient atrophy, inflammation or distortion to prevent confusion of the Barrett's mucosa with normal, but this is not a reliable criterion. Due to great variability in the normal squamocolumnar junction we regard with skepticism the diagnosis of Barrett's esophagus based on the identification of gastric cardiac mucosa within 2 cm proximal to the LES but are more confident with gastric fundic glands containing parietal and chief cells. Equivocal results may require additional multiple biopsies from different levels.

Several groups of children are at risk of developing Barrett's esophagus from GER due to esophageal dysfunction. Children with esophageal atresia and tracheoesophageal fistula often have abnormal lower esophageal sphincter function, GER, and esophagitis which, if not

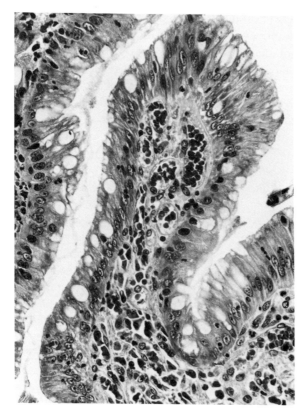

Fig. 11. Barrett's esophagus, specialized columnar type. Goblet cells are abundant in the surface epithelium of this patient. The chronic inflammation in the lamina propria is often observed in Barrett's esophagus. HE. ×625.

treated, can lead to the development of a Barrett's esophagus [15]. Developmentally or mentally delayed children often have esophageal dysmotility predisposing them to esophagitis and Barrett's esophagus. Four of our patients with cystic fibrosis had Barrett's esophagus found during evaluation for chronic abdominal pain thought to be secondary to peptic ulcer disease. We identified Barrett's esophagus in 2 children with leukemia, one with a bone marrow transplant, when they were endoscoped because of heartburn, odynophagia, and a clinical diagnosis of infectious esophagitis. The sequelae of Barrett's esophagus in children remains uncertain. Fewer than 10% of adults with Barrett's esophagus develop adenocarcinoma in the lower one-third of the esophagus [37, 38] leading to the recommendation for yearly endoscopy and biopsy to detect dysplastic changes. We have not identified cytologic atypia with Barrett's esophagus in children. Universally accepted clinical approaches to the management of Barrett's esophagus in children have not yet been formulated. It is important to accurately diagnose and follow children with Barrett's esophagus in order to clarify its course and significance in this age group.

Persistent Embryonic Columnar Epithelium and
Congenital Heterotopic Gastric Epithelium in the Esophagus

Although not often encountered in a mucosal biopsy, persistent embryonic columnar epithelium and congenital heterotopic gastric epithelium enter into the differential diagnosis of Barrett's esophagus. During the first half of intrauterine life, ciliated stratified columnar epithelium lines the esophagus (fig. 12). At approximately 20 weeks' gestation, transformation to stratified squamous epithelium begins at midesophagus and simultaneously proceeds proximally and distally to cover the entire esophagus by the 25th week of embryonic life [39] although occasionally delayed or incomplete, leaving a strip or patch of superficial columnar epithelium within the stratified squamous epithelium. The columnar epithelium is usually identified incidentally at autopsy, particularly in prematurely born infants and not usually after several weeks of age, when it is apparently replaced by squamous epithelium. Columnar epithelium is most likely to persist at the proximal or distal ends of the esophagus, the last sites replaced in normal development [40]. With our neonatal autopsy routine of obtaining two esophageal sections per case, one longitudinally through the gastroesophageal junction and one cross-section through the neck block, we occasionally encounter persistent embryonic columnar epithelium (fig. 13) although systematic search may reveal it more commonly [41].

Heterotopic gastric mucosa including columnar surface epithelium and lamina propria with well-developed gastric glands is almost exclusively found in the upper esophagus, usually as one or several small patches in the post-cricoid region. Heterotopic gastric mucosa is almost always asymptomatic and has been encountered incidentally at autopsy in infants, children and adults at all ages [42, 43]. The gross appearance of the patches has been likened to small erosions or shallow ulcers. The gastric

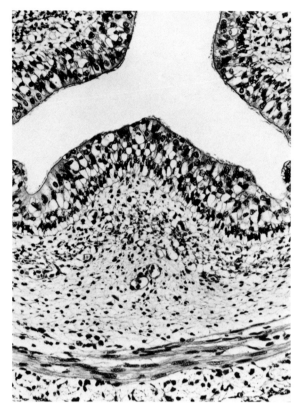

Fig. 12. Esophageal mucosa from a human fetus of thirteen weeks gestational age with ciliated stratified columnar epithelium and lack of glands within the lamina propria. HE. ×25.

glands are usually of cardiac type but may be fundic with parietal and chief cells. We found heterotopic gastric mucosa in only 1 patient, (fig. 14) a 15-year-old girl with abdominal pain and nausea due to peptic ulcer disease. A patch of salmon-pink mucosa was identified by endoscopy just below the cricopharyngeus surrounded by normal appearing esophageal mucosa. Biopsies of this area revealed heterotopic gastric mucosa which apparently was not responsible for her symptoms.

Willis [43] regarded heterotopic gastric mucosa in the esophagus as abnormal differentiation of the pluripotential embryonic columnar lining. In this sense, persistent embryonic columnar epithelium and the more

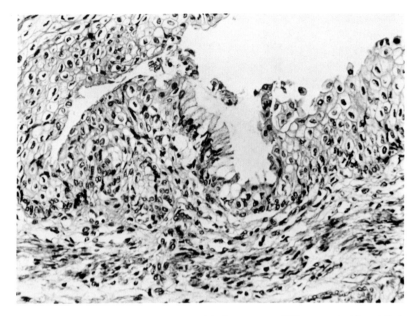

Fig. 13. Persistent embryonic columnar epithelium, center. This was an incidental finding near the esophagogastric junction in a one-day-old infant of 30 weeks' gestation. HE. ×250.

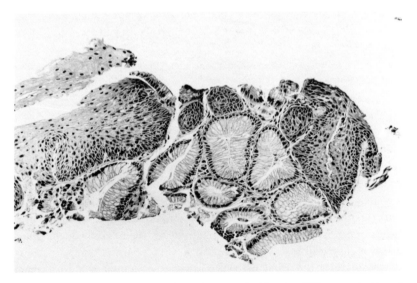

Fig. 14. Heterotopic gastric mucosa from the post-cricoid region. This was an incidental finding during endoscopy for evaluation of peptic ulcer disease. HE. ×130.

elaborately developed gastric heterotopias represent altered differentiation. Both persistent embryonic epithelium and heterotopic gastric epithelium have caused confusion with Barrett's esophagus and delayed acceptance of Barrett's esophagus in children. Barrett's esophagus affects the lower one-third of the esophagus in continuity with the gastroesophageal junction while heterotopic gastric epithelium occupies the upper (postcricoid) esophagus. Barrett's esophagus, with transformation of the entire mucosa including superficial columnar epithelium and a complex gastric glandular layer bears little resemblance to normal embryonic esophagus or to persistent embryonic columnar epithelium, except for the shared feature of superficial columnar epithelium. Heterotopic postcricoid gastric epithelium may resemble junctional and fundic types of Barrett's epithelium histologically, but the location and clinical setting are quite different. Heterotopic post-cricoid gastric epithelium is usually asymptomatic, whereas Barrett's esophagus accompanies symptoms of gastroesophageal reflux.

Infectious Esophagitis

Infectious esophagitis rarely affects nonhospitalized and nonimmunosupressed children, but occasionally must be distinguished from the much more common reflux esophagitis. In children with cancer, bone marrow transplant, or with prolonged antibiotic therapy, esophageal symptoms are more likely due to infection than to gastroesophageal reflux.

Herpes simplex Esophagitis

Herpes simplex causes esophagitis in immunosuppressed and debilitated patients [44] and otherwise normal individuals as well [45, 46]. Esophageal involvement by herpes may be isolated or occur as part of a widespread infection. Isolated herpes esophagitis is the more common occurrence. In an autopsy series of adults with herpes infections, the esophagus was affected in 89%, in 73% the esophagus was the only organ involved [47]. Because of the frequent use of a nasogastric tube, esophageal trauma may predispose to the development of herpes esophagitis. In otherwise healthy children, herpetic esophagitis may occur alone or accompany herpetic gingivo-stomatitis. In immunosuppressed children, herpes infection is often a reactivation of previously encountered herpes virus infection.

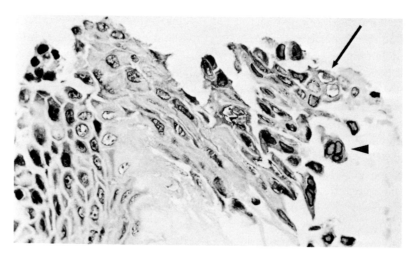

Fig. 15. Epithelial changes in herpes simplex esophagitis in a nonimmunosuppressed child include spongiosis and nuclear pyknosis (left). Cowdry type A inclusions (full arrow) and multinucleated herpes giant cells (Cowdry, type B inclusions, arrowhead) are present at the margin of an ulcer (right). HE. ×700.

Endoscopically herpetic esophagitis usually presents with multiple small, well-circumscribed ulcers located anywhere throughout the length of the esophagus. With very extensive involvement, usually identified at autopsy, the distal esophagus may have confluent circumferential ulceration. Ulcers contain nonspecific necrotic and inflammatory debris occasionally infected secondarily with bacteria or fungi. Herpes virus inclusions, whose demonstration is key to the diagnosis, are found at ulcer margins.

The histologic diagnosis of herpes simplex esophagitis [44, 48] can often be suspected from low magnification microscopic observation of a severe degree of ulceration and necrosis not often encountered in reflux esophagitis. At higher magnification (fig. 15) the epithelial cellular changes are characteristic of herpes simplex infection: spongiosis, ballooning degeneration and bland necrosis, often with epithelial thinning or ulceration. Intraepithelial polymorphonuclear leukocytes are often abundant, in contrast to their sparcity in reflux esophagitis. Other inflammatory cells are also abundant in epithelium and lamina propria. At high magnification, some nuclei of infected cells have a ground-glass appearance; other nuclei are pale with margination of chromatin and prominent nucleoli.

Histologic diagnosis of herpes requires identification of the character-istic inclusions: Cowdry type A eosinophilic intranuclear inclusions with a halo or Cowdry type B, homogeneous ground-glass nuclear inclusions which are often in multinucleated herpes giant cells. These are best found in ulcer margins with typical cellular alterations, necrosis, and neutrophilic infiltrate of herpetic infection. At times, however, even an optimally ob-tained specimen will fail to show characteristic cellular changes or inclu-sions. The number of inclusions varies widely from rare to plentiful and are best found at autopsy in large tissue sections. Identification of inclu-sions in small mucosal biopsies may be difficult.

In 3 nonimmunosuppressed children with herpes esophagitis, 2 pa-tients with herpes simplex virus cultured from endoscopically obtained tis-sue had no inclusion bodies in mucosal specimens taken at the same endo-scopic session. All 3 children showed abundant intraepithelial eosinophils. Only one of the three children had previous esophageal symptoms consi-dered due to GER prior to developing herpes esophagitis. The signifi-cance of intraepithelial eosinophils in the other 2 children is uncertain. Perhaps viral esophagitis results in loss of integrity of the lower esophageal sphincter, resulting in reflux.

Fungal Esophagitis

Fungal infection of the esophagus is usually due to Candida species, and usually limited to immunosuppressed or debilitated, long-term hospi-tal patients treated with antibiotics, children with mucocutaneous can-didiasis, and infants maintained for a long time in neonatal intensive care units. Candida esophagitis has been reported in adults superimposed on esophagitis due to GER [49], but we have not encountered this complica-tion of GER in children. Endoscopically, candida usually appears in the lowest one-third of the esophagus, occasionally more diffuse, as white plaques, with or without surrounding hyperemia and ulcerations. Mild in-fection may have a nonspecific appearance [50–52].

The histologic appearance may vary with the extent of the infection and the vigor of the inflammatory response. Candidal plaques (fig. 16) or pseudomembranes consist of heaped up epithelial and inflammatory de-bris and fibrin, admixed with typical yeast and pseudohyphal forms, appa-rent on hematoxylin and eosin stain, but accentuated with Gomori's methenamine silver or periodic acid-Schiff stains. Adjacent and underly-ing mucosa contains acute and chronic inflammation in those who can muster an inflammatory response. Eosinophils are not increased. Shallow

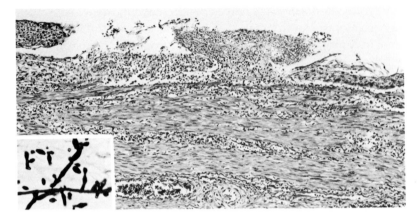

Fig. 16. Candida esophagitis, with ulceration and plaque at center and epithelial remnants at sides. The plaque is composed of fibrin and epithelial and inflammatory debris. Organisms are not visible at this magnification, but pseudohyphae and yeast forms were visualized (inset) in plaque and mucosa with Gomori's methenamine silver stain. HE. ×11. Inset: Gomori's methenamine silver. ×400.

ulcers may also be present. As with herpetic ulcers, bacteria may overgrow the ulcer bed.

Less commonly, aspergillus may cause esophagitis [53, 54], particularly in patients with cancer undergoing chemotherapy. Clinical and pathologic findings are similar to those of esophageal candidiasis, including ulcerations, plaques and necrosis.

Both candida and aspergillus have the potential for deep invasion, at times penetrating through the esophageal muscularis resulting in mediastinitis, disseminated infection, tracheoesophageal fistula [53], and erosion into large mediastinal blood vessels.

Cytomegalovirus Esophagitis

Cytomegalovirus (CMV) rarely causes isolated esophagitis. More commonly, esophagitis is part of disseminated CMV viremia or infection throughout the gastrointestinal tract [55–57]. All reported patients with CMV esophagitis have had altered immune status. The gross pathologic features of CMV esophagitis include focal ulcerations and plaques. Microscopically, characteristic inclusion bodies accompany nonspecific inflam-

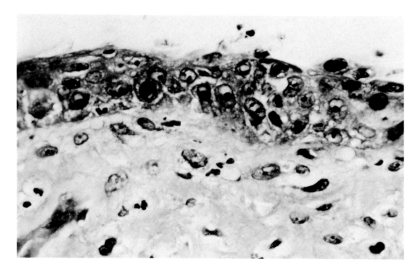

Fig. 17. Esophageal epithelial atypia in a child on high dose methotrexate regimen for lymphoblastic lymphoma. HE. ×700.

mation. Although most cases are identified at autopsy, occasional cases have been diagnosed by mucosal biopsy [58, 59]. There were no cases among our biopsies. We found CMV esophagitis in a child with acute myeloblastic leukemia who had a bone marrow transplant and died of systemic CMV infection.

The Esophagus in Immunosuppressed Patients

Children receiving cancer chemotherapy and the recipients of a bone marrow transplant form the second largest group after GER in whom esophageal biopsy is performed in our hospital. These patients are prone to esophageal problems because of their chemotherapy, immunosuppression, radiation therapy and, debilitation. Most antineoplastic drugs interfere with cell replication. Due to the rapid replication time of esophageal and gastrointestinal epithelium, these sites are particularly sensitive to antineoplastic drugs. Esophageal response to chemotherapy varies widely with differences in drugs, dose schedule, and individual factors. Acute effects include edema, inflammation and ulceration during administration of the agent, epithelial nuclear atypia and changes in mitotic activity (either increased or decreased) (fig. 17).

Patients with cancer undergoing chemotherapy are susceptible to esophageal disease from a variety of sources: drug toxicity, graft versus host disease (GVHD), infection from Candida, herpes virus or cytomegalovirus. Polymicrobial infection may occur with multiple fungi, or a fungus plus a virus. Esophagitis may be the portal of entry for disseminated infection in these patients.

Chemotherapy and repeated episodes of esophagitis may predispose to a chronic, noninfectious esophagitis resulting in esophageal dysmotility and GER. Two of our patients with Barrett's esophagus had cancer, a relationship noted by others [60].

Following allogeneic bone marrow transplant, the esophagus may be the site of GVHD. Changes in the esophageal mucosa identified by biopsy in acute GVHD are similar to those in skin: vacuolization and lymphocytic infiltration of the basal layer of epithelium, eosinophilic bodies in epithelium, and inflammatory cell infiltration of the lamina propria [61]. Esophageal disease is more likely in chronic GVHD, 3 or more months posttransplant [60], when findings include submucosal fibrosis associated with mucosal inflammation and ulceration. Esophageal GVHD may occur at any level of the esophagus, but more commonly in the proximal half.

Conclusion

Very few pediatric subspecialists depend on the surgical pathologist as does the gastroenterologist. Mucosal biopsy evaluation is key to the diagnosis in many gastrointestinal diseases. In esophageal disorders particularly, endoscopy and mucosal biopsy have become part of the accepted diagnostic approach. Endoscopic findings may be nonspecific or, as in the case of reflux esophagitis, actually misleading. In addition to establishing an initial diagnosis, mucosal biopsy can be used to determine response to therapy. Most esophageal biopsies in children relate to gastroesophageal reflux, but there are other applications as well. The procedure has a role in monitoring patients with Barrett's esophagus. Mucosal biopsy will often demonstrate an organism or show viral inclusion bodies in infectious esophagitis. Biopsy is especially helpful in oncology patients, with their myriad of esophageal problems. Considering that esophageal biopsies were not performed in children until approximately 10 years ago, it is impressive how frequently they are done today, and how important they have become in patient management.

References

1 Whitehead, R.: Normal appearances in oesophageal biopsy specimens; in Mucosal biopsy of the gastrointestinal tract; 3rd ed., pp. 3–5 (Saunders, Philadelphia 1985).

2 Weinstein, W.C.; Bogoch, E.R.; Bowes, K.L.: The normal esophageal mucosa: a histological reappraisal. Gastroenterology 68: 40–44 (1975).

3 Behar, J.; Sheahan, D.C.: Histologic abnormalities in reflux esophagitis. Archs Path. 99: 387–391 (1975).

4 Ismail-Beigi, F.; Horton, P.F.; Pope, C.E.: Histological consequences of gastroesophageal reflux in man. Gastroenterology 58: 163–174 (1970).

5 Goldman, H.; Antonioli, D.A.: Mucosal biopsy of the esophagus, stomach and proximal duodenum. Human Pathol. 13: 423–448 (1982).

6 Herbst, J.J.: Gastroesophageal reflux. J. Pediat. 98: 859–870 (1981).

7 Euler, A.R.; Ament, M.E.: Gastroesophageal reflux in children. Clinical manifestations, diagnosis, pathophysiology and therapy. Pediat. Ann. 5: 678–689 (1976).

8 Herbst, J.J.; Meyers, W.F.: Gastroesophageal reflux in children. Adv. Pediat. 28: 159–186 (1981).

9 Weissbluth, M.: Gastroesophageal reflux. A review. Clin. Pediat. 20: 7–14 (1981).

10 Rothstein, F.C.; Halpin, T.C.: High incidence of pulmonary symptoms in infants evaluated for esophageal disease. Ann. Otol. Rhinol. Lar. 89: 450–453 (1980).

11 Euler, A.R.; Byrne, W.J.; Ament, M.E.: Recurrent pulmonary disease in children. A complication of gastroesophageal reflux. Pediatrics, Springfield 63: 47–51 (1979).

12 Biller, J.A.; Winter, H.S.; Grand, R.J.; Allred, E.N.: Are endoscopic changes predictive of histologic esophagitis in children? J. Pediat. 103: 215–218 (1983).

13 Bendig, D.W.; Seilheimer, D.K.; Wagner, M.L.; Ferry, G.D.; Harrison, G.M.: Complications of gastroesophageal reflux in patients with cystic fibrosis. J. Pediat. 100: 536–540 (1982).

14 Thomas, D.; Rothberg, R.M.; Lester, L.A.: Cystic fibrosis and gastroesophageal reflux in infancy. Am. J. Dis. Child. 139: 66–67 (1985).

15 Winter, H.S.; Madara, J.L.; Stafford, R.J.; et al.: Delayed acid clearance and esophagitis after repair of esophageal atresia. Gastroenterology 80: 1317 (1981).

16 Benjamin, B.; Pohl, B.; Bale, P.M.: Endoscopy and biopsy in gastroesophageal reflux in infants and children. Ann. Otol. 89: 443–445 (1980).

17 Whitehead, R.: Gastro-oesophageal reflux and oesophagitis; in Mucosal biopsy of the gastrointestinal tract; 3rd ed., pp. 6–17 (Saunders, Philadelphia 1985).

18 Richter, J.E.; Castell, D.O.: Gastroesophageal reflux: Pathogenesis, diagnosis and therapy. Ann. intern. Med. 97: 93–103 (1982).

19 Winter, H.S.; Madara, J.L.; Stafford, R.J.; Grand, R.J.; Quinlan, J.; Goldman, H.: Intraepithelial eosinophils. A new diagnostic criterion for reflux esophagitis. Gastroenterology 83: 818–823 (1982).

20 Geboes, L.; Desmet, V.; Vantrappen, G.: Esophageal histology in the early stage of gastroesophageal reflux. Archs Pathol. Lab. Med. 103: 205 (1979).

21 Katz, A.J.; Goldman, H.; Grand, R.J.: Gastric mucosal biopsy in eosinophilic (allergic) gastroenteritis. Gastroenterology 73: 705–709 (1977).

22 Cello, J.P.: Eosinophilic gastroenteritis – a complex disease entity. Am. J. Med. 67: 1097–1104 (1979).

23   Dobbins, J.W.; Sheahan, D.G.; Behar, J.: Eosinophilic gastroenteritis with esophageal involvement. Gastroenterology *72:* 1312–1316 (1977).

24   Jona, J.Z.; Belin, R.P.; Burke, J.A.: Eosinophilic infiltration of the gastrointestinal tract in children. Am. J. Dis. Child. *130:* 1136–1139 (1976).

25   Haggitt, R.C.; Meissner, W.H.: Crohn's disease of the upper gastrointestinal tract. Am. J. clin. Path. *59:* 613–622 (1973).

26   Miller, L.J.; Thistle, J.L.; Payne, W.S.; et al.: Crohn's disease involving the esophagus and colon. Case report. Mayo Clin. Proc. *52:* 35–38 (1977).

27   LiVolsi, V.A.; Jaretzki, A.: Granulomatous esophagitis. A case of Crohn's disease limited to the esophagus. Gastroenterology *64:* 313–319 (1973).

28   Bozymski, E.M.; Herlihy, K.J.; Orlando, R.C.: Barrett's esophagus. Ann. intern. Med. *97:* 103–107 (1982).

29   Messian, R.A.; Hermos, J.A.; Robbins, A.H.; et al.: Barrett's esophagus: Clinical review of 26 cases. Am. J. Gastroent. *69:* 458–466 (1978).

30   Mossberg, S.M.: The columnar-lined esophagus (Barrett syndrome). An acquired condition. Gastroenterology *50:* 671–676 (1966).

31   Barrett, N.R.: Chronic peptic ulcer of the oesophagus and oesophagitis. Br. J. Surg. *38:* 175–182 (1950).

32   Bremner, C.G.; Lynch, V.P.; Ellis, F.H.: Barrett's esophagus: congenital or acquired? An experimental study of esophageal mucosal regeneration in the dog. Surgery *68:* 209–216 (1970).

33   Wong, J.; Finckh, E.S.: Heterotopia and ectopia of gastric epithelium by mucosal wounding in the rat. Gastroenterology *60:* 279–287 (1971).

34   Dahms, B.B.; Rothstein, F.C.: Barrett's esophagus in children. A consequence of chronic gastroesophageal reflux. Gastroenterology *86:* 318–323 (1984).

35   Rothstein, F.C.; Dahms, B.B.: Barrett's esophagus in children; in Spechler, Goyal, Barrett's esophagus: pathophysiology, diagnosis and management (Elsevier, New York, in press, 1985).

36   Paull, A.; Trier, J.S.; Dalton, M.D.; Camp, R.C.; Loeb, P.; Goyal, R.J.: The histologic spectrum of Barrett's esophagus. New Engl. J. Med. *295:* 476–480 (1976).

37   McDonald, G.B.; Brand, D.L.; Thorning, D.R.: Multiple adenomatous neoplasms arising in columnar-lined (Barrett's) esophagus. Gastroenterology *72:* 1317–1321 (1977).

38   Berenson, M.M.; Riddell, R.H.; Skinner, D.B.; Freston, J.W.: Malignant transformation of esophageal columnar epithelium. Cancer *41:* 554–561 (1978).

39   Johns, B.A.E.: Developmental changes in the oesophageal epithelium in man. J. Anat. *86:* 431–442 (1952).

40   Enterline, H.; Thompson, J.: The normal esophagus – embryology, structure and function; in Pathology of the esophagus, pp. 1–21 (Springer, New York 1984).

41   Rector, L.E.; Connerley, M.L.: Aberrant mucosa in the esophagus in infants and children. Archs Pathol. Lab. Med. *31:* 285–294 (1941).

42   Taylor, A.L.: The epithelial heterotopias of the alimentary tract. J. Path. Bact. *30:* 415–449 (1927).

43   Willis, R.A.: Developmentally heterotopic tissues; in The borderland of embryology and pathology, pp. 306–340 (Butterworth, London 1958).

44   Nash, G.; Ross, J.S.: Herpetic esophagitis, a common cause of esophageal ulceration. Human Pathol. *5:* 339–345 (1974).

45 Depew, W.T.; Prentice, R.S.A.; Beck, I.T.; et al.: Herpes simplex esophagitis in a healthy subject. Am. J. Gastroent. 63: 381–385 (1977).

46 Bastian, J.F.; Kaufman, I.A.: Herpes simplex esophagitis in a healthy 10-year-old boy. J. Pediat. 100: 426–427 (1982).

47 Buss, D.H.; Scharyj, M.: Herpesvirus infection of the esophagus and other visceral organs in adults. Am. J. Med. 66: 457–562 (1979).

48 McKay, J.S.; Day, D.W.: Herpes simplex oesophagitis. Histopathology 7: 409–420 (1983).

49 Lefkowitz, M.; Elsar, J.L.; Levine, R.J.: Candida infection complicating peptic esophageal ulcer. Archs intern. Med. 113: 672–675 (1964).

50 Kodsi, B.E.; Wickremesinghe, P.C.; Kozinn, P.J.; Iswara, K.; Goldberg, P.K.: Candida esophagitis. A prospective study of 27 cases. Gastroenterology 71: 715–719 (1976).

51 Mathieson, R.; Dutta, S.K.: Candida esophagitis. Dig. Dis. Sci. 28: 365–370 (1983).

52 Scott, B.B.; Jenkins, D.: Gastro-oesophageal candidiasis. Gut 23: 137–139 (1982).

53 Obrecht, W.F.; Richter, J.E.; Olympio, G.A.; Gelfand, D.W.: Tracheoesophageal fistula. A serious complication of infectious esophagitis. Gastroenterology 87: 1174–1179 (1984).

54 Young, R.C.; Bennett, J.E.; Vogel, C.L.; et al.: Aspergillosis. The spectrum of the disease in 98 patients. Medicine 49: 147–170 (1970).

55 Wong, T.; Warner, N.E.: Cytomegalic inclusion disease in adults. Archs Path. 74: 403–422 (1962).

56 Freeman, H.J.; Shnitka, T.K.; Piercey, J.R.A.; Weinstein, W.M.: Cytomegalovirus infection of the gastrointestinal tract in a patient with late onset immunodeficiency syndrome. Gastroenterology 73: 1397–1403 (1977).

57 Peterson, P.K.; Balfour, H.H.; Marker, S.C.; et al.: Cytomegalovirus disease in renal allograft recipients. A prospective study of the clinical features, risk factors and impact on renal transplantation. Medicine 59: 283–300 (1980).

58 Allen, J.I.; Silvis, S.E.; Sumner, H.W.; McClain, C.J.: Cytomegalic inclusion disease diagnosed endoscopically. Dig. Dis. Sci. 26: 133–135 (1981).

59 St.-Onge, G.; Bezahler, G.H.: Giant esophageal ulcer associated with cytomegalovirus. Gastroenterology 83: 127–130 (1982).

60 McDonald, G.B.; Sullivan, K.M.; Schuffler, M.D.; et al.: Esophageal abnormalities in chronic graft-versus-host disease in humans. Gastroenterology 80: 914–921 (1981).

61 Slavin, R.E.; Woodruff, J.M.: The pathology of bone marrow transplantation; in Somners, Pathology annual, vol. 9, pp. 291–344 (Appleton-Century-Crofts, New York 1974).

B.B. Dahms, MD, Departments of Pathology and Pediatrics, Case Western Reserve University, School of Medicine and Rainbow Babies and Children's Hospital, Cleveland, OH 44106 (USA)

Perspect. pediatr. Pathol., vol. 11, pp. 124–151 (Karger, Basel 1987)

Gastroesophageal Reflux and Esophagitis in Infants and Children[1]

Pamela A. Groben[a], *Gene P. Siegal*[a, c], *Mitchell D. Shub*[b], *Martin H. Ulshen*[b], *Frederic B. Askin*[a]

[a]Divisions of Surgical and [c]Oncologic Pathology, Department of Pathology and the [b]Division of Pediatric Gastroenterology, Department of Pediatrics, University of North Carolina School of Medicine, Chapel Hill, N.C.

Introduction

Gastroesophageal reflux (GER) commonly occurs in infants and young children, often manifest simply by 'spitting up' or transient vomiting episodes, but also by persistent, serious and potentially life-threatening complications. A recent increased interest in the histologic diagnosis of esophagitis in children with GER concomitant with new diagnostic techniques to identify significant GER has accompanied an increased interest in the surgical management of these children, particularly those at risk for complications. Histologically, intraepithelial eosinophils may be an early and specific marker of prolonged acid reflux in children with GER [1].

Criteria for the diagnosis of abnormal or 'pathologic' reflux have been defined through the use of several diagnostic studies. The acid reflux (Tuttle) test, the overnight intraesophageal pH probe and the barium esophagram are the most widely used studies [2–4]. We have evaluated the endoscopic biopsies of a group of 33 infants less than 2 years of age with

[1] This investigation was supported in part by a Dean's Fund Award. Dr. Groben is a Regular Clinical Fellow and Dr. Siegal is a Junior Faculty Clinical Fellow of the American Cancer Society (CF No. 5733, JFCF No. 739).

radiologic or pH probe evidence of abnormal GER for the presence of intraepithelial eosinophils and other histopathologic evidence of eso-phagitis. The children in our series were compared with a group of age matched control infants to determine the significance of the histologic findings. Our studies suggest that reproducible criteria for the histologic diagnosis of esophagitis can be obtained even in very young infants. Fur-thermore, in infants with clinically significant GER, not only is esophagitis common, but the severity of inflammation may increase after 6 months of age. Histologic esophagitis may frequently occur in the absence of gross endoscopic findings.

Esophageal Physiology

The distal esophagus has a zone of increased intraluminal pressure but not a distinct anatomic sphincter. The intraabdominal position of the distal esophagus, the angle at which the esophagus enters the stomach and the ligamentous attachments aid this lower esophageal sphincter (LES) to pre-vent free reflux of gastric contents into the esophagus in normal individu-als [5]. GER is very common in infants and usually improves spontane-ously with age. This may be a function of gradual maturation in lower esophageal sphincter pressure in normal infants during the first 6 weeks of age [6, 7].

The role of LES pressure in preventing GER remains controversial [8, 9, 10]. The basal LES pressure of normal controls overlaps with chil-dren with radiologically proven GER [10, 11]. Transient, inappropriate re-laxation of the LES [12], a short LES segment [9, 10], transient increase in abdominal pressures [13] and delayed gastric emptying [14] may play a role in the pathogenesis of GER [15].

The relationship between hiatus hernia and GER is likewise contro-versial. Children with hiatus hernia are at increased risk for GER [16–18], but few children with GER have hiatus hernia [10, 19]. The severity of re-flux does not relate to the size of the hernia and clinical improvement in GER can occur despite a persistent hiatus hernia [10, 20]. A hiatus hernia need not cause reflux by raising LES pressure, since patients with symp-toms of GER may have low LES pressures [21]. In the natural history of GER with hiatus hernia, 60% of children were symptom free by 18 months to 2 years, 90–95% were symptom free by age 4, and 5% developed stric-tures or died of complications [22].

Clinical Manifestations and Diagnosis

The varied symptoms and clinical manifestation of GER [5, 23–25] include effortless emesis or regurgitation as the most common finding, occurring in approximately 80% of affected children at birth or within the first 2 months of life [24, 26]. Some infants may have projectile vomiting associated with delayed gastric emptying or pyloric stenosis [15, 27]. Persistent vomiting may result in failure to thrive with poor weight gain [24, 27]. Other common manifestations include pulmonary complications including aspiration pneumonia (12%), and anemia, melena and hematemesis (38%). Severe esophagitis with erosion of the surface mucosa results in esophageal bleeding and, less commonly, a stricture of the esophagus [28].

As an important cause of chronic pulmonary disease in children [29–33], GER has been related to chronic asthma and recurrent pneumonia with improvement or resolution of pulmonary symptoms following successful therapy for GER [29, 31]. Forty-seven percent of steroid-dependent asthmatic children [32] and 6% of children with recurrent obstructive bronchitis had GER [30].

Recurrent apnea in infants and children has been attributed to GER with aspiration [24, 34]. This process can cause radiographic findings similar to bronchopulmonary dysplasia. Although apnea is usually sleep related, an 'awake apnea syndrome' and 'near miss' sudden infant death syndrome [36–39] has also been associated with GER [35]. Apnea has been demonstrated in close temporal relationship to GER by some [34] but not by others [40–41]. In several infants less than 6 months of age with recurrent respiratory arrest and GER, surgical fundoplication resulted in resolution of both the GER and the apneic episodes [36], supporting an etiologic role for reflux in the apneic attacks. Others, however, have not demonstrated a temporal relationship between apneic episodes and GER episodes under controlled conditions [40, 41]. GER seems a likely factor in triggering apnea in a small group of infants, perhaps as many as 10% of patients with near-miss SIDS [5].

GER in children may cause symptoms which adults with GER rarely have. Symptoms suggesting a CNS disorder include dystonia, developmental retardation, dysphagia, irritability and seizure-like activity [42], an unusual head cocking posture (Sandifer's syndrome) [43–45], rumination in which food is regurgitated and rechewed [23, 46], and a protein-losing enteropathy with finger clubbing [47].

In some children at increased risk for GER, the primary abnormality may mask the symptoms of reflux. Of institutionalized mentally retarded children, 11% had significant reflux [48]; an even higher percentage was seen in patients with neurologic disorders [49]. GER is also common in children following repair of esophageal atresia and is associated with abnormal motility of the distal esophagus [50–52]. Some children with congenital heart disease and neurologic impairment have GER [53], and their respiratory symptoms may be due to reflux rather than to the heart disease.

Barium Esophagram

Although the sensitivity of barium esophagram has been reported to be low (50%), the method is widely available and provides useful anatomic information [2, 54]. The presence of hiatus hernia, esophageal stricture, adequacy of gastric emptying, pyloric stenosis or other anatomic abnormalities as well as esophageal function and peristalsis can be studied [5, 17, 23, 55–58].

Recently, McCauley et al. [4] reported a standardized approach to a radiographic evaluation of GER in children in which the extent of reflux is graded. Age-related criteria include an acceptable amount of reflux in children [18]. Using the standardized approach of McCauley et al. [4], the sensitivity of the standardized barium esophagram as compared to the 24-hour pH probe was 86%, but the specificity was only 21% [59].

Severe reflux demonstrated radiographically may correlate with the complications of reflux (fig. 1). Radiologic signs of mucosal alteration correlate well with severe histologic esophagitis or ulceration [58]. Major reflux identified radiologically has a strong statistical correlation with pulmonary disease [60]. As many as 100% of those infants and children who eventually require surgical correction of GER have demonstrable reflux on barium esophagram [4, 26, 61]. A detailed clinical history suggesting GER and significant reflux on barium esophagram using strict and age related criteria are adequate to make the diagnosis in some cases, but equivocal or negative examinations require additional tests.

Scintigraphy

Gastroesophageal (GE) scintiscanning is a convenient method to detect GER in children [62–65] using a small amount of ^{99m}Tc sulfur colloid and scan of the esophageal area (fig. 2). The method is noninvasive, does not require sedation, exposes the infant to less radiation than a barium

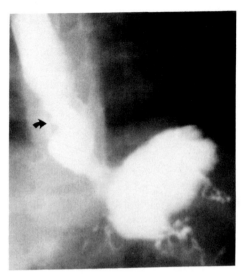

Fig. 1. An upper gastrointestinal barium study demonstrating severe esophagitis with an esophageal ulcer (arrow).

esophagram and permits study over a prolonged length of time. If radioactivity is detected in the lung during delayed imaging, pulmonary aspiration can be confirmed [66, 67]. Delayed gastric emptying associated with GER can also be detected [68].

The reported sensitivity of this method varies from 56.6% of the children with positive acid reflux (Tuttle) tests [54] to 75–79% [56, 69]. With a specificity of 71–93% [59, 69], the scintiscan is inferior to barium studies for demonstrating GE anatomy [70] but combination of the two tests increases sensitivity [54].

Intraesophageal pH Monitoring: Acid Reflux Test

With the acid reflux or Tuttle test as modified for use in infants and children [2, 71, 72], a calculated volume of 0.1 N HCl is instilled into the stomach through a nasogastric tube which is then removed. With the pH probe positioned above the distal 1/5 of the esophagus, the patient is placed in several different positions and abdominal compression is applied if spontaneous reflux is not noted. Two or more episodes of reflux, defined as a drop of pH to less than 4, are considered abnormal. This test has a 90–97% correlation with symptomatic GER [54, 73]. Using the 24-hour in-

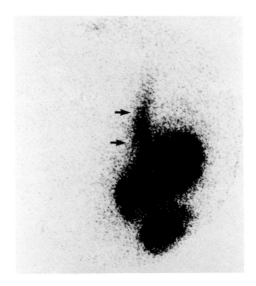

Fig. 2. A gastroesophageal scintiscan demonstrating esophageal reflux (arrows).

traesophageal pH probe (see below) as a standard, the acid reflux test was 100% specific and 77% sensitive [11], with a 20% rate of false-positive tests in an asymptomatic control group of adults [74].

The acid reflux test has the disadvantages of not being a physiologic procedure [75, 76], of requiring exogenous acid instillation into the stomach, and the sedation of infants.

Extended pH Monitoring

Extended pH monitoring eliminates most of the disadvantages of the acid reflux test and is considered to be more sensitive [3, 75–80]. With the pH electrode in the esophagus as in the acid reflux test, the patient is given a liquid or normal diet and the intraesophageal pH is continuously monitored for 18–24 h. The position of the infant and information as to whether the child is awake, asleep, eating, crying or having respiratory difficulties are recorded every 30 min (fig. 3). Reflux is defined as a fall in pH to less than 4 for at least 15 s [3]. The parameters measured and quantitated include: (1) the number of reflux episodes; (2) the number of reflux episodes of more than 5 min duration; (3) the duration of the longest reflux episode; (4) the percentage of the total amount of time the pH is less than

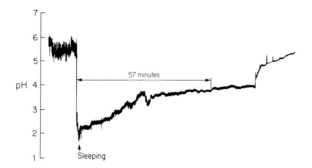

Fig. 3. Extended intraesophageal pH probe study demonstrating a 57 minute episode of reflux.

4 [3]. From a total pH score, control children can be clearly separated from those with GER. Frequently, the control population has 'physiologic' reflux in the first 2 h after a meal. Reflux, when it occurred in the control group, was usually seen in children who were awake or upright. Control children rarely refluxed when sleeping supine although this was a common occurrence in children with symptomatic GER. The prone position has been associated with fewer but more prolonged reflux episodes [80].

Since prolonged contact between the esophageal mucosa and gastric acid has been correlated with the severity of esophagitis [77, 80, 81], a new parameter, clearance time in pH probe monitoring studies has been introduced [76]. It measures the time required for the pH to return to prereflux values after a reflux episode, but has not shown consistent correlation between the severity of esophagitis and clearance time [83]. Prolonged nocturnal episodes of reflux have been associated with pulmonary aspiration or respiratory symptoms [67, 82].

Use of prolonged pH monitoring identified three postprandial patterns of GER in children less than 2 years of age [79, 84]: continuous, discontinuous and mixed. The discontinuous pattern of reflux was associated in some cases with delayed gastric emptying and with the spontaneous resolution of reflux usually by 10 months of age in 63% of cases. Continuous or mixed patterns of reflux were associated with a low incidence of spontaneous resolution and a high (50%) chance of eventual need of surgical intervention.

Extended pH monitoring provides the most sensitive and specific test available to detect GER and, despite occasional errors, forms the standard to evaluate other tests [11, 85]. A 3-hour pH monitoring test [83, 86], and pH monitoring by telemetry have also been described [87].

Esophageal Manometry

The LES pressure in control patients overlaps with those of GER. Manometry and biopsy can be performed simultaneously in adults. However, this is usually not possible in children. Thus, in different age groups, different sites may be biopsied if the endoscopist does not sample the grossly most abnormal region. Normal children generally do not have a LES pressure less than 10 mm Hg; a sphincter with a pressure less than 10 mm Hg can be considered incompetent [86, 88]. A very low LES pressure (less than 6 mm Hg) has been associated with esophagitis [54]. Whether the lower pressure causes or results from severe esophagitis is unclear. Manometry is useful in identifying motility disturbances [6, 89] and in localizing the LES for accurate placement of the pH electrode for monitoring or for biopsy.

Endoscopic Biopsy and the Histology of Esophagitis

As a term, 'reflux esophagitis' has unfortunately been used interchangeably with gastroesophageal reflux to describe the symptom complex related to reflux. Almost all infants and children reflux at some time; not all reflux is necessarily abnormal. GER which produces symptoms or complications is abnormal and can usually be uncovered by one of the aforementioned diagnostic methods. Endoscopy and biopsy are performed to assess one of the complications of reflux, i.e. esophagitis [90, 91]. Biopsy is always necessary, even if the endoscopic findings are normal, although only a proportion of patients with abnormal or symptomatic GER have histologic esophagitis. Recently, Biller et al. [91] found that 30% of children with normal endoscopic findings had histologic esophagitis. The presence of histologic esophagitis may also help to confirm the presence of reflux when other diagnostic methods have been equivocal. Endoscopy and biopsy help evaluate response to therapy, provide prognostical data, and help assess the need for surgical therapy to prevent or to treat stricture formation.

Because the gross and microscopic changes of esophagitis may occur in a patchy distribution, results of pH testing, radiologic examination, manometry, endoscopy and morphologic studies often do not correlate well with each other [54, 58, 88, 91].

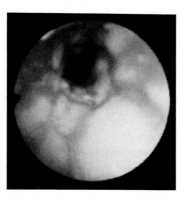

Fig. 4. Endoscopic view of severe esophagitis with mucosal erosions, nodularity and a fixed stricture.

Clinical Data

To more clearly define the histologic criteria for esophagitis in infants less than 25 months of age, we compared the biopsies in a group of infants with clinical reflux to a control population of the same age. GER was diagnosed in the study group of 33 consecutive infants (less than 25 months of age) between 1979 and 1983 at North Carolina Memorial Hospital (NCMH). Children were excluded if they had an associated neoplasm, disseminated infection, or failed to have clinical GER. The diagnosis of GER was made following positive test results: (1) Tuttle test; (2) overnight intraesophageal pH monitoring; (3) barium esophagram [92]. All patients had esophageal endoscopy [93]. By gross examination, ulceration, nodularity or friability identified esophagitis (fig. 4). Erythema alone was not a criterion of endoscopic esophagitis [94, 95]. All patients had biopsies from the mid-esophagus with grasp forceps (site 2); 27 patients had additional biopsies from a more distal location (site 1), and all biopsies were cephalad to the distal 1/5 of the esophagus.

Only 6 (18%), of our 33 patients, had gross esophagitis (table I). Of the 27 others, 14 patients (52%) had histologic esophagitis. The study patients were evaluated initially for symptoms of recurrent vomiting (22 patients), for failure to thrive (6 patients), apneic episodes (7 patients), or chronic respiratory symptoms (4 patients). The mean age of the study patients was 9 months; 64% were male and 36% were female.

The control population, retrieved from the files of the Office of the North Carolina State Medical Examiner, was composed of 19 infants (12

Table I. Esophageal histology in 6 patients with gross endoscopic evidence of esophagitis[1]

Age, months	1 or more EOS/HPF	20 PMNs/HPF	Ulceration
5[2]	0	0	0
11	+	+	+
12	+	0	0
14	+	+	+
17	+	+	+
20	+	0	+
Total	5/6 (83%)	3/6 (50%)	4/6 (67%)

[1] Data from either site.
[2] Mild friability only.

girls, 7 boys) less than 25 months of age (mean 9 months) who died within 12 h, suffering lethal trauma. None of the infants in the control population had been intubated and most died immediately. Cases of possible sudden infant death syndrome and of the caustic ingestion were excluded. GER was not mentioned in the clinical records of any of the control patients. Esophageal tissue was obtained from above the distal 1/4 of the esophagus.

Study Methods

Hematoxlin and eosin stained slides of formalin-fixed tissue were examined independently in all cases by 3 pathologists, who did not know the clinical histories, endoscopic and special study findings, or each other's results. Cell counts were obtained for intraepithelial and stromal eosinophils and polymorphonuclear leukocytes (PMNs) in every case. The one high power field (400×) with the greatest number of neutrophils or eosinophils in the epithelium and stroma was used for the absolute cell count. The sections were also examined for intraepithelial and stromal lymphoid cells, intraepithelial 'wiggly' cells, basal zone hyperplasia (greater than 1/5), papillary lengthening (greater than 2/3), ulceration, and Barrett's epithelium (see below). Intraepithelial 'wiggly' cells were defined as the angulated, molded mononuclear cells found among the squamous epithelial cells. At the completion of the study the cases were reviewed and difference between observers resolved in a consensus conference.

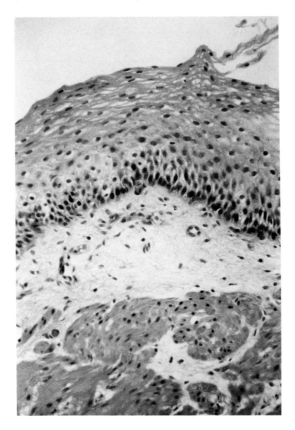

Fig. 5. In a full thickness section of a normal esophagus, the thin basal cell layer lies at the interface between the mucosa and submucosal stroma. HE. ×250.

Interobserver differences were present in less than 10% of the total number of variables.

Chi-square tests of homogeneity were used to study the proportions of individual variables within the study group and control population to determine if the populations were significantly different. The Fisher-Irwin exact test for 2×2 tables was used for groups of less than 5. The two biopsy sites in the patient group were also compared to identify any difference between the sites with respect to intraepithelial and stromal polymorphonuclear leukocytes and eosinophils.

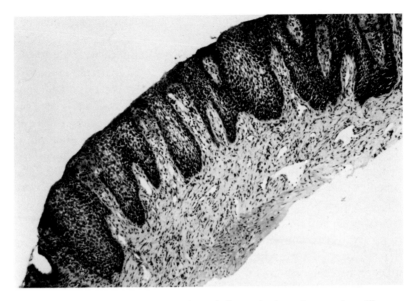

Fig. 6. Esophagitis. The basal cell layer is hyperplastic and stromal papillae are lengthened so that they almost reach the epithelial surface. HE. ×100.

Pathology

Basal Zone Hyperplasia and Papillary Lengthening

Basal cell hyperplasia of the esophageal mucosal epithelium and increased stromal papillary length have been used to identify esophagitis [97] (fig. 5, 6), but with variations in criteria of diagnosis, selection of biopsy site, type of biopsy (pinch vs. suction), and the method of measurement [96–100].

Thickening of the basal cell layer to greater than 1/5 of the total epithelial thickness and a papillary length of greater than 3/5 of the mucosal thickness are the most commonly used criteria. Because basal zone hyperplasia and papillary lengthening occur normally in the distal 2.5 cm of the esophagus [101], biopsies from this area are to be avoided. Specimens are taken above the distal 5 cm in infants and children [1, 100]. Basal zone hyperplasia or papillary lengthening may be estimated from standard brightfield microscopy without the use of an occular reticle, but precise criteria [96–98] require at least two papillae per section with a clearly defined central core of lamina propria. The basal layer is measured from the basal lamina to the point where the nuclei are separated by a distance equal to their diameter.

Johnson et al. [98] found a direct correlation between both percent papillary lengthening and percent basal zone hyperplasia and an intraesophageal pH less than 4. A statistically significant percent papillary extension occurred in patients with abnormal 24-hour composite pH scores, although the 'normal' group had higher values than the criterion used as abnormal (50%) by others [96, 98]. Basal zone hyperplasia and papillary lengthening evaluated by morphometric techniques [100] revealed no significant difference between normal and GER, or with pH function tests with the data of Johnson et al. [98]. An arbitrary value of 60% papillary lengthening provides a significant difference between control patients and reflux patients. These studies point out the problems in using these criteria to make a diagnosis in an individual patient. Difficulties are compounded with small pinch biopsy specimens or by inter and intra-observer variation [99]. Basal zone hyperplasia or papillary lengthening were not evaluable in over 70% of our group of 33 patients.

Vascular Dilatation

As a diagnostic criterion for esophagitis, marked dilatation of the capillaries in the papillae of the epithelium occurred in 83% of patients with clinical GER, as compared to only 10% of controls, a statistically significant difference [102, 103]. Since the passage of the endoscope could cause similar vascular changes, we do not use isolated vascular dilation as a diagnostic criterion.

Lymphoid Infiltrates

Lymphocytes and plasma cells normally occupy the lamina propria and squamous epithelium of the esophagus [96, 97, 100]. There was no statistical difference between our control group and the pediatric patient population with respect to the presence or absence of mononuclear cells in the epithelium or stroma (fig. 7).

We found no statistical difference in incidence of 'wiggly' cells, although they appear to be increased in esophagitis (fig. 8). The nature of 'wiggly' cells remains unknown. Using monoclonal antibodies, the mononuclear cells in the squamous epithelium of controls and patients with gastroesophageal reflux [104], identified as cytotoxic T lymphocytes and Langerhans' cells, were increased in number in esophagitis. Helper T cells and B lymphocytes were present chiefly in the lamina propria in both groups.

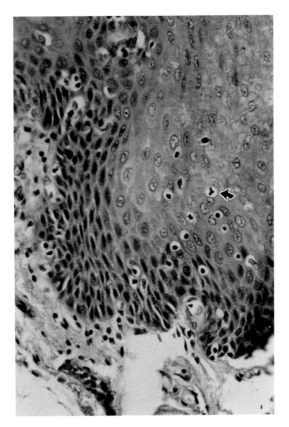

Fig. 7. Lymphoid cells of no diagnostic importance interdigitate among the mucosal epithelial cells. One polymorphonuclear leukocyte (PMN) lies within the epithelium (arrow). HE. ×400.

Tissue Eosinophils

Polymorphonuclear leukocytes and eosinophils within the esophageal mucosa are markers for esophagitis [1, 99, 100, 105, 106]. Of patients with prolonged acid reflux, 50% had intraepithelial eosinophils, an uncommon finding in control patients. Even a single eosinophil correlates with abnormal acid clearance by 24-hour pH probe studies and with basal zone hyperplasia. Eosinophils are highly specific but relatively insensitive for detecting delayed acid clearance. Since eosinophils appear in half the patients under the age of 2 in the absence of basal zone hyperplasia, eosinophils may be an earlier marker for esophageal injury than basal

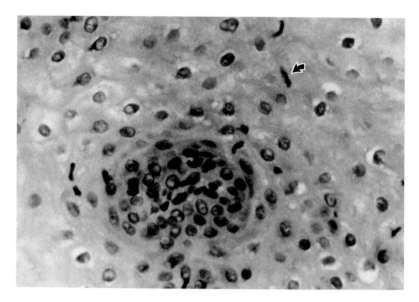

Fig. 8. The angulated 'wiggly' cells (arrows) lie between squamous epithelial cells and in cross sections of papillae (center). Wiggly cells appear to be increased in esophagitis but are also present in normal patients. HE. ×400.

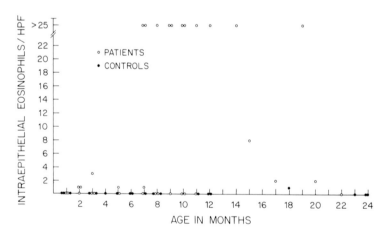

Fig. 9. Representation of the number of intraepithelial eosinophils/HPF in children segregated by age in months at the time of initial biopsy. Nineteen of 33 infants with GER but only 1 of the control children had one or more intraepithelial eosinophils.

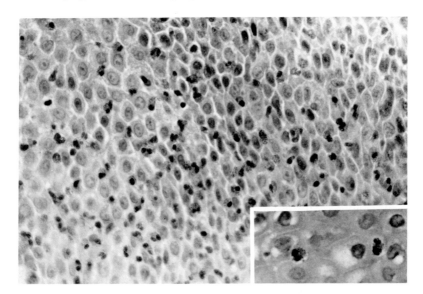

Fig. 10. Intraepithelial eosinophils with their characteristic bilobated nuclei and cyto-plasmic granules are prominent in esophagitis. HE. Original magnification ×250. Inset: HE. ×400.

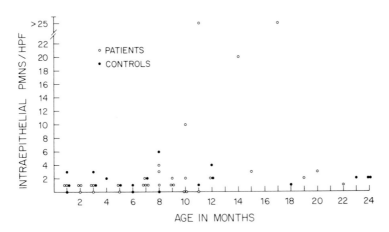

Fig. 11. Polymorphonuclear cells/HPF tabulated according to patient's age in months show no significant difference between the control and patient groups because of the few cells in both groups.

zone hyperplasia or papillary lengthening and may identify patients at risk for more severe complications of acid reflux, i.e. ulceration or stricture [1].

We strongly support the use of intraepithelial eosinophils as a marker of esophagitis in young children. Of our patients with GER, 58% had intraepithelial eosinophils as compared to less than 5% of control patients (fig. 9, 10), a highly significant difference (p=0.0001). One or more intraepithelial eosinophils per biopsy is generally adequate for the diagnosis of esophagitis even in young infants; all of our patients less than 7 months of age had at least 1–3 eosinophils per HPF. One 'positive' control patient had a single intraepithelial eosinophil.

Of adults with esophagitis, 30–60% had eosinophils in the lamina propria, but so did 10–33% of controls [96, 100, 107]. Of our 33 children, eosinophils in the lamina propria were statistically significant for one biopsy site (p=0.033) but of only borderline significance for the other site (p=0.0675). The difference between the sites probably has no biological significance as they are from the same region of the esophagus. As we interpret the data, eosinophils within the lamina propria may be significant for the diagnosis of esophagitis, but not at the same level of certainty as intraepithelial eosinophils.

Tissue Polymorphonuclear Leukocytes

PMNs are markers for esophageal inflammation in adults and are absent in the controls [96, 100]. In our quantitation of intraepithelial PMNs, most controls had rare (1–3) intraepithelial PMNs with an average of 1.63 PMNs/HPF, negating a statistical difference between the GER patients and control group (p=0.5), (fig. 11). We found no value which would separate the two groups statistically because of the small number of study patients with more than rare (1–3) PMNs/HPF.

Rare intraepithelial PMNs (1–3/HPF) are common in normal children and are not useful as markers for early esophagitis. Few of our patients had 4 or more PMNs/HPF and most of these patients also had intraepithelial eosinophils. The diagnosis was questionable in 1 patient with 4 intraepithelial PMNs and no eosinophils. Most patients with greater than 4 PMNs/HPF had numerous (>20 PMNs/HPF) PMNs often in association with eosinophils (table II). A large number of PMNs often accompanies severe esophagitis or ulceration [96, 99, 107] (fig. 12). Of our 5 patients with ulceration at either site 1 or 2, 60% had 20 or more intraepithelial PMNs/HPF (table III). We do not accept 1–3 intraepithelial PMNs/HPF in

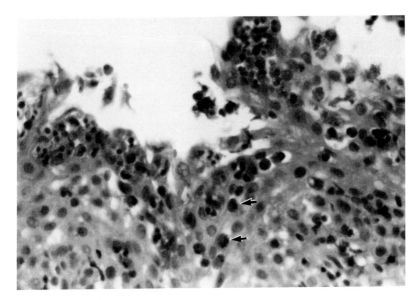

Fig. 12. Severe esophagitis characterized by numerous intraepithelial eosinophils (arrows), polymorphonuclear leukocytes and microscopic surface erosions. HE. ×400.

Table II. Esophageal histology in 5 patients with greater than 4 intraepithelial PMNs/HPF[1]

Age, months	Intraepithelial PMNs	Intraepithelial eosinophils	Ulceration	Endoscopic abnormalities
8	4	0	o	o
10	10	TNTC	o	o
11	TNTC	TNTC	o	+
14	20	TNTC	+	+
17	TNTC	2	+	+

TNTC=Too numerous to count (>20/HPF).
o=No; +=yes.
[1] Data from site 2.

the absence of eosinophils as diagnostic of esophagitis although greater than 20 intraepithelial PMNs/HPF indicates moderate or severe esophagitis. Although probably indicative of esophagitis, 4–19 intraepithelial PMNs/HPF has indeterminate clinical significance and requires additional diagnostic criteria (table IV).

Table III. Esophageal histology in 5 patients with histologic ulceration[1]

Age, months	Number of eosinophils	Number of PMNs
9	TNTC	1
11	22	TNTC
14	TNTC	20
17	2	TNTC
20	3	15

[1] Ulceration present at either site 1 or site 2.

Table IV. Histologic criteria for diagnosis of esophagitis in infants

Absolute[1]
1 One or more intraepithelial eosinophils/HPF
2 Greater than 20 intraepithelial PMNs/HPF
3 Ulceration

Indeterminate-probably diagnostic
1 Basal zone hyperplasia <20%[2]
2 Papillary lengthening <60%[2]
3 Stromal eosinophils
4 4–19 intraepithelial PMNs/HPF

Not diagnostic – contributory
1 Dilated capillaries in stromal papillae
2 Increase number of intraepithelial 'wiggly cells'
3 Stromal PMNs

Not helpful
1 One-three intraepithelial PMNs/HPF
2 Lymphoid infiltrates

[1] With proper clinical setting, see text.
[2] Not evaluable in 70% of our grasp biopsies.

Barrett's Esophagus

In adults, Barrett's esophagus (a columnar epithelium-lined eso-phagus) accompanies chronic gastroesophageal reflux as an acquired and perhaps premalignant condition in about 11% of patients [108, 109]. In children (8 months to 19 years) with gastroesophageal reflux, 13% had Barrett's esophagus established histologically [110]. Three of our 33 in-fants aged 2 to 7 months (9%) had Barrett's esophagus (fig. 13), all diag-

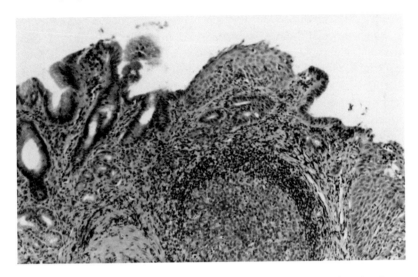

Fig. 13. Barrett's epithelium from an infant with esophagitis showing junctional type gastric epithelium within the esophagus. HE. ×250.

nosed by biopsies from site 1 (more distal) but above the Z line (junction of gastric and esophageal mucosa). Each patient had 1 of the 3 types of epithelia described by Paull et al. [111]. The youngest infant had only a tiny fragment of intestinal type epithelium, the other 2 infants had atrophic gastric fundic epithelium. All of our infants with Barrett's esophagus had histologic features of esophagitis (intraepithelial eosinophils). No patient had Barrett's epithelium without other histologic evidence of esophagitis, suggesting that Barrett's is acquired and can develop in a short time.

Treatment

Medical and surgical treatment regimes aimed at reducing reflux and preventing its complications consist initially of thickened small feedings and an upright, prone, or 30° elevated prone position, with results of therapy monitored by pH assessment [112–114]. Bethanechol, a cholinergic drug which increases the LES pressure and increases lower esophageal motility, has been effective in infants [115–117] when other medical regimes fail. Metoclopramide improves LES tone, symptomatic GER and gastric emptying and does not increase gastric acid secretion [118–120].

Surgery is indicated for the approximate 15% of symptomatic children in whom medical therapy is unsuccessful [61]. The indications for surgery are similar in most series [26, 27, 49, 121–127]. The exceptions to a medical trial are children with esophageal stricture or life-threatening episodes of apnea or 'near miss' SIDS. Other indications for surgery include recurrent aspiration pneumonia, intractable emesis, failure to thrive, bleeding, apnea and severe esophagitis refractory to medical therapy but not necessarily Barrett's esophagus. Complications of GER vary with different age groups. Life-threatening apnea, and severe failure to thrive with growth retardation usually present in the first year of life [124, 125, 127]. With rare exceptions severe esophagitis with strictures affects older infants and children [124, 127, 128].

Nissen fundoplication, the most widely used and successful surgical treatment for GER [121–125, 127–131], provides symptomatic relief in over 90% of the children [122, 124, 127, 131, 133–136] with very low operative mortality. Experience with other surgical procedures is less extensive [26, 132]. Complications of the surgery in some patients include an inability to burp or vomit (i.e. the 'gas bloat' syndrome) after fundoplication [127]. Control of GER in some patients may not result in control of respiratory symptoms, apnea or failure to thrive, especially in those patients with associated neurologic disorders, seizures, cardiac defects or multiple anomalies [49, 126, 133].

Acknowledgement

The authors thank Ms. B. Nunn for typing the manuscript and its many revisions. Preliminary work from this study has previously been published in abstract form [Siegal et al.: Lab. Invest. 50: 12P, 1984; Shub et al.: Gastroenterology 86: 1251, 1984]. The authors also thank Eliana Marques and the Department of Biostatistics, University of North Carolina School of Public Health for the statistical analysis.

References

1   Winter, H.S.; Madars, J.L.; Stafford, R.J.; Grand, R.J.; Quinlan, J.E.; Goldman, H.: Intraepithelial eosinophils. A new diagnostic criterion for reflux esophagitis. Gastroenterology 83: 818–823 (1982).
2   Euler, A.R.; Ament, M.E.: Detection of gastroesophageal reflux in the pediatric-age patient by esophageal intraluminal pH probe measurement (Tuttle test). Pediatrics, Springfield 60: 65–68 (1977).

3   Jolley, S.G.; Johnson, D.G.; Herbst, J.J.; Pena, A.; Garnier, R.: An assessment of
    gastroesophageal reflux in children by extended pH monitoring of the distal esophagus.
    Surgery *84:* 16–24 (1978).

4   McCauley, R.G.; Darling, D.B.; Leonidas, J.C.; Schwartz, A.M.: Gastroesophageal
    reflux in infants and children. A useful classification and reliable physiologic technique
    for its demonstration. Am. J. Roentg. *130:* 47–50 (1978).

5   Herbst, J.J.: Gastroesophageal reflux. J. Pediat. *98:* 859–870 (1981).

6   Boix-Ochoa, J.B.: Diagnosis and management of gastroesophageal reflux in children.
    Surg. A. *13:* 123–137 (1981).

7   Boix-Ochoa, J.B.; Canals, J.: Maturation of the lower esophagus. J. pediat. Surg. *11:*
    749–756 (1976).

8   Euler, A.R.; Ament, M.E.: Value of esophageal manometric studies in the gas-
    troesophageal reflux of infancy. Pediatrics, Springfield *59:* 58–61 (1977).

9   Herbst, J.J.; Book, L.S.; Johnson, D.G.; Jolley, S.: The lower esophageal sphincter in
    gastroesophageal reflux in children. J. clin. Gastroenterol. *1:* 119–123 (1979).

10 Moroz, S.P.; Espinoza, J.; Cumming, W.A.; Diamant, N.E.: Lower esophageal
    sphincter function in children with and without gastroesophageal reflux. Gastroenterol-
    ogy *71:* 236–241 (1976).

11 Euler, A.R.; Byrne, W.J.: Twenty-four hour esophageal intraluminal pH probe test-
    ing. A comparative analysis. Gastroenterology *80:* 957–961 (1981).

12 Werlin, S.L.; Dodds, W.J.; Hogan, W.J.; Arndorfer, R.C.: Mechanisms of gastro-
    esophageal reflux in children. J. Pediat. *97:* 244–249 (1980).

13 Dodds, W.J.; Dent, J.; Hogan, W.J.; Helm, J.F.; Hauser, R.; Patel, G.K.; Egide,
    M.S.: Mechanisms of gastroesophageal reflux in patients with reflux esophagitis. New
    Engl. J. Med. *307:* 1547–1552 (1982).

14 Hillemeier, A.C.; Lange, R.; McCalum, R.; Seashore, J.; Gryboski, J.: Delayed gas-
    tric emptying in infants with gastroesophageal reflux. J. Pediat. *98:* 190–193 (1981).

15 Rode, H.; Cywes, S.; Davies, M.R.: The phreno-pyloric syndrome in symptomatic gas-
    troesophageal reflux. J. pediat. Surg. *17:* 152–157 (1982).

16 Carre, I.J.: Disorders of the oro-pharynx and esophagus; in Anderson, et al., Pediatric
    gastroenterology, pp. 33–79 (Blackwell, Oxford 1975).

17 Darling, D.B.; Fisher, J.H.; Gellis, S.S.: Hiatal hernia and gastroesophageal reflux in
    infants and children. Analysis of the incidence in North American children. Pediatrics,
    Springfield *54:* 450–455 (1974).

18 Cleveland, R.H.; Kushner, D.C.; Schwartz, A.N.: Gastroesophageal reflux in chil-
    dren. Results of a standardized fluoroscopic approach. Am. J. Roentg. *141:* 53–56
    (1983).

19 Vanderhoof, J.A.; Ament, M.E.: Letter. Hiatal hernia and gastroesophageal reflux. J.
    Pediat. *88:* 693–695 (1976).

20 Carcassone, M.; Bensonsson, A.; Aubert, J.: The management of gastroesophageal re-
    flux in infants. J. pediat. Surg. *8:* 575–585 (1973).

21 Cohen, S.; Harris, C.P.: Does hiatus hernia affect competence of the lower esophageal
    sphincter? New Engl. J. Med. *284:* 1053 (1971).

22 Carre, I.J.: The natural history of the partial thoracic stomach (hiatus hernia) in chil-
    dren. Archs Dis. Childh. *34:* 344–353 (1959).

23 Herbst, J.J.; Meyers, W.F.: Gastroesophageal reflux in children. Adv. Pediat. *28:* 159–
    186 (1981).

24 Weissbluth, M.: Gastroesophageal reflux. A review. Clin. Pediat. *20:* 7–14 (1981).

25 Euler, A.R.; Ament, M.E.: Gastroesophageal reflux in children. Clinical manifestations, diagnosis, pathophysiology, and therapy. Pediat. A. *5:* 678–689 (1976).

26 Johnson, D.G.; Herbst, J.J.; Oliveros, M.A.; Stewart, D.R.: Evaluation of gastroesophageal reflux surgery in children. Pediatrics, Springfield *59:* 62–68 (1977).

27 Randolph, J.G.; Lilly, J.R.; Anderson, K.D.: Surgical treatment of gastroesophageal reflux in infants. Ann. Surg. *180:* 479–489 (1974).

28 Fonkalsrud, E.W.; Ament, M.E.; Byrne, W.J.; Rachelefsky, G.S.: Gastroesophageal fundoplication for the management of reflux in infants and children. J. thorac. cardiovasc. Surg. *76:* 655–664 (1978).

29 Berquist, W.E.; Rachelefsky, G.S.; Kadden, M.; Siegel, S.C.; Katz, R.M.; Fonkalsrud, E.W.; Ament, M.E.: Gastroesophageal reflux-associated recurrent pneumonia and chronic asthma in children. Pediatrics, Springfield *68:* 29–35 (1981).

30 Danus, O.; Casar, C.; Larrain, A.; Pope, C.E.: Esophageal reflux. An unrecognized cause of recurrent obstructive bronchitis in children. J. Pediat. *89:* 220–224 (1976).

31 Euler, A.R.; Byrne, W.J.; Ament, M.E.; Fonkalsrud, E.W.; Strobel, C.T.; Siegel, S.C.; Katz, R.M.; Rachelefsky, G.S.: Recurrent pulmonary disease in children. A complication of gastroesophageal reflux. Pediatrics, Springfield *63:* 47–51 (1979).

32 Shapiro, G.G.; Christie, D.L.: Gastroesophageal reflux in steroid dependent asthmatic youths. Pediatrics, Springfield, *63:* 207–212 (1979).

33 Nelson, H.S.: Gastroesophageal reflux and pulmonary disease. J. Allergy clin. Immunol. *73:* 547–556 (1984).

34 Herbst, J.J.; Minton, S.D.; Book, L.S.: Gastroesophageal reflux causing respiratory distress and apnea in newborn infants. J. Pediat. *95:* 763–768 (1979).

35 Spitzer, A.R.; Boyle, J.T.; Tuchman, D.N.; Fox, W.W.: Awake apnea associated with gastroesophageal reflux. A specific clinical syndrome. J. Pediat. *104:* 200–205 (1984).

36 Leape, L.L.; Holder, T.M.; Franklin, J.D.; Amoury, R.A.; Ashcraft, K.W.: Respiratory arrest in infants secondary to gastroesophageal reflux. Pediatrics, Springfield *60:* 924–928 (1977).

37 MacFadyen, U.M.; Hendry, G.M.; Simpson, H.: Gastroesophageal reflux in near-miss sudden infant death syndrome or suspected recurrent aspiration. Archs Dis. Childh. *58:* 87–91 (1983).

38 Jeffery, H.E.; Reid, I.; Rahilly, P.; Read, D.J.: Gastro-esophageal reflux in 'near miss' sudden infant death syndrome or suspected recurrent aspiration. Archs Dis. Childh. *58:* 87–91 (1983).

39 Herbst, J.J.; Book, L.S.; Bray, P.F.: Gastroesophageal reflux in the 'near miss' sudden infant death syndrome. J. Pediat. *92:* 73–75 (1978).

40 Walsh, J.K.; Farrell, M.K.; Keenan, W.J.; Lucas, M.; Kramer, M.: Gastroesophageal reflux in infants: relation to apnea. J. Pediat. *99:* 197–201 (1981).

41 Ariagno, R.L.; Guilleminault, C.; Baldwin, R.; Owen-Boeddiker, M.: Movement and gastroesophageal reflux in awake term infants with 'near miss' SIDS, unrelated to apnea. J. Pediat. *100:* 894–897 (1982).

42 Bray, P.F.; Herbst, J.J.; Johnson, D.G.; Book, L.S.; Ziter, F.A.; Condon, V.R.: Childhood gastroesophageal reflux. Neurologic and psychiatric syndromes mimicked. J. Am. med. Ass. *237:* 1342–1345 (1977).

43 Kinsborne, M.: Hiatus hernia with contortions of the neck. Lancet *i:* 1058 (1964).

44 Snyder, C.H.: Paroxymal torticollis in infancy. Am. J. Dis. Child. *117:* 458–460 (1969).

45 Sutcliffe, J.: Torsion spasms and abnormal posture in children with hiatus hernia, Sandifer's syndrome. Prog. pediat. Radiol. *2:* 190–197 (1969).

46 Herbst, J.J.; Friedland, G.W.; Zboralske, F.F.: Hiatal hernia and 'rumination' in infants and children. J. Pediat. *78:* 261–265 (1971).

47 Herbst, J.J.; Johnson, D.G.; Oliveros, M.A.: Gastroesophageal reflux with protein-losing enteropathy and finger clubbing. Am. J. Dis. Child. *130:* 1256–1258 (1976).

48 Feldman, W.: Gastroesophageal reflux in retarded children (Letter). Pediatrics, Springfield *94:* 850–851 (1979).

49 Jolley, S.G.; Herbst, J.J.; Johnson, D.G.; Matlak, M.E.; Book, L.S.: Surgery in children with gastroesophageal reflux and respiratory symptoms. J. Pediat. *96:* 194–198 (1980).

50 Parker, A.F.; Christie, D.L.; Cahill, J.L.: Incidence and significance of gastroesophageal reflux following repair of esophageal atresia and tracheoesophageal fistula and the need for anti-reflux procedures. J. pediat. Surg. *14:* 5–8 (1979).

51 Orringer, M.B.; Kirsh, M.M.; Sloan, H.: Long-term esophageal function following repair of esophageal atresia. Ann. Surg. *186:* 436–443 (1977).

52 Shermeta, D.W.; Whitington, P.F.; Seto, D.S.; Haller, J.A.: Lower esophageal sphincter dysfunction in esophageal atresia. Nocturnal regurgitation and aspiration pneumonia. J. pediat. Surg. *12:* 871–876 (1977).

53 Weesner, K.M.; Rosenthal, A.: Gastroesophageal reflux in association with congenital heart disease. Clin. Pediat. *22:* 424–426 (1983).

54 Arasu, T.S.; Wyllie, R.; Fitzgerald, J.F.; Franken, E.A.; Siddiqui, A.R.; Lehman, G.A.; Eigen, H.; Grosfeld, J.L.: Gastroesophageal reflux in infants and children. Comparative accuracy of diagnostic methods. J. Pediat. *96:* 798–803 (1980).

55 Darling, D.B.: Hiatal hernia and gastroesophageal reflux in infancy and childhood. Analysis of the radiologic findings. Am. J. Roentg. Rad. Ther. nucl. Med. *123:* 724–736 (1975).

56 Steiner, G.M.: Gastroesophageal reflux, hiatus hernia and the radiologist, with special reference to children. Br. J. Radiol. *50:* 164–174 (1977).

57 Swischuk, L.E.; Hayden, C.K., Jr.; Van-Callie, B.D.: Mega-aeroesophagus in children: a sign of gastroesophageal reflux. Radiology *141:* 73–76 (1981).

58 Darling, D.B.; McCauley, R.G.; Leape, L.L.; Ramenofsky, M.L.; Bhan, I.; Leonidas, J.C.: The child with peptic esophagitis. A correlation of radiologic signs with esophageal pathology. Radiology *145:* 673–676 (1982).

59 Siebert, J.J.; Byrne, W.J.; Culer, A.R.; Latture, T.; Leach, M.; Campbell, M.: Gastroesophageal reflux – the acid test. Scintigraphy or the pH probe? Am. J. Roentg. *140:* 1087–1090 (1983).

60 Darling, D.B.; McCauley, R.G.; Leonidas, J.C.; Schwartz, A.M.: Gastroesophageal reflux in infants and children. Correlation of radiological severity and pulmonary pathology. Radiology *127:* 735–740 (1978).

61 Randolph, J.: Experience with the Nissen fundoplication for correction of gastroesophageal reflux in infants. Ann. Surg. *198:* 579–584 (1983).

62 Fisher, R.S.; Malmud, L.S.; Roberts, G.S.; Lobis, I.F.: Gastroesophageal (GE) scintiscanning to detect and quantitate GE reflux. Gastroenterology *70:* 301–307 (1976).

63 Heyman, S.; Kirkpatrick, J.A.; Winger, H.S.; Treves, S.: An improved radionuclide method for the diagnosis of gastroesophageal reflux and aspiration in children (milk scan). Radiology *131:* 479–482 (1979).

64 Rudd, T.G.; Christie, D.L.: Demonstration of gastroesophageal reflux in children by radionuclide gastroesophagography. Radiology *131:* 483–486 (1979).

65 Sty, J.R.; Starshak, R.J.: The role of radionuclide studies in pediatric gastrointestinal disorders. Semin. nucl. Med. *12:* 156–172 (1982).

66 Jona, J.Z.; Sty, J.R.; Glicklich, M.: Simplified radioisotope technique for asessing gastroesophageal reflux in children. J. pediat. Surg. *16:* 114–117 (1981).

67 Chernow, B.; Johnson, L.F.; Janowitz, W.R.; Castell, D.O.: Pulmonary aspiration as a consequence of gastroesophageal reflux. Dig. Dis. Sci. *24:* 839–844 (1979).

68 Seibert, J.J.; Byrne, W.J.; Euler, A.R.: Gastric emptying in children: unusual patterns detected by scintigraphy. Am. J. Roentg. *141:* 49–51 (1983).

69 Blumhagen, J.D.; Rudd, T.G.; Christie, D.L.: Gastroesophageal reflux in children: radionuclide gastroesophagography. Am. J. Roentg. *135:* 1001–1004 (1980).

70 Roberts, C.C.; Herbst, J.J.; Jolley, S.G.; Johnson, D.G.: Evaluation of tests for gastroesophageal reflux in patients operated on for tracheoesophageal fistula. Pediat. Res. *14:* 509 (1980).

71 Tuttle, S.G.; Grossman, M.I.: Detection of gastroesophageal reflux by simultaneous measurement of intraluminal pressure and pH. Proc. Soc. exp. Biol. Med. *98:* 225–227 (1958).

72 Christie, D.L.: The acid reflux test for gastroesophageal reflux. J. Pediat. *94:* 78–81 (1979).

73 Benz, L.J.; Hootkin, L.A.; Margulies, S.; Donner, M.W.; Cauthorne, R.T.; Hendrix, T.R.: A comparison of clinical measurements of gastroesophageal reflux. Gastroenterology *62:* 1–5 (1972).

74 DeMeester, T.R.; Johnson, L.F.: The evaluation of objective measurements of gastroesophageal reflux and their contribution to patient management. Surg. Clins N. Am. *56:* 39–53 (1976).

75 Soundheimer, J.M.: Continuous monitoring of distal esophageal pH. A diagnostic test for gastroesophageal reflux in infants. J. Pediat. *96:* 804–807 (1980).

76 Koch, A.; Gass, R.: Continuous 20–24 hour esophageal pH-monitoring in infancy. J. pediat. Surg. *16:* 109–113 (1981).

77 Johnson, L.F.; DeMeester, T.R.: Twenty-four hour pH monitoring of the distal esophagus. Am. J. Gastroent. *62:* 325–332 (1974).

78 Hill, J.L.; Pelligrini, C.A.; Burrington, J.D.; Reyes, H.M.; DeMeester, T.R.: Technique and experience with 24-hour esophageal pH monitoring in children. J. pediat. Surg. *12:* 877–887 (1977).

79 Jolley, S.G.; Herbst, J.J.; Johnson, D.G.; Book, L.S.; Matlak, M.E.; Condon, V.R.: Patterns of postcibal gastroesophageal reflux in symptomatic infants. Am. J. Surg. *138:* 946–950 (1979).

80 Boix-Ochoa, J.; Lafuenta, J.M.; Gil-Vernet, J.M.: Twenty-four hour esophageal pH monitoring in gastroesophageal reflux. J. pediat. Surg. *15:* 74–78 (1980).

81 Stanciu, C.; Bennett, J.R.: Oesophageal acid clearing. One factor in the production of reflux esophagitis. Gut *15:* 852–857 (1974).

82 Jolley, S.G.; Herbst, J.J.; Johnson, D.G.; Matlak, M.E.; Book, L.S.: Esophageal pH monitoring during sleep identifies children with respiratory symptoms from gastroesophageal reflux. Gastroenterology *80:* 1501–1506 (1981).

83 Reyes, H.M.; Ostrovsky, E.; Radhakrishnan, J.: Diagnostic accuracy of a three hour continuous intraluminal pH monitoring of the lower esophagus in the evaluation of gastro-esophageal reflux in infancy. J. pediat. Surg. *17:* 625–631 (1982).

84   Jolley, S.G.; Johnson, D.G.; Herbst, J.J.; Matlak, M.E.: The significance of gastroesophageal reflux patterns in children. J. pediat. Surg. *16:* 859–865 (1981).

85   Roberts, C.C.; Herbst, J.J.; Jolley, S.G.; Johnson, D.G.: Evaluation of tests for gastroesophageal reflux in patients operated on for tracheoesophageal fistula. Pediat. Res. *14:* 509 (1980).

86   Reyes, H.M.; Ostrovsky, E.: Diagnosis and treatment of gastroesophageal reflux in infants and children. Surg. A. *15:* 61–71 (1983).

87   Falor, W.H.; Chang, B.; White, H.A.; Kraus, J.M.; Taylor, B.; Hansel, J.R.; Kraus, F.C.: Twenty-four hour esophageal pH monitoring by telemetry. Cost-effective use in outpatients. Am. J. Surg. *142:* 514–516 (1981).

88   Behar, J.; Biancani, P.; Sheahan, D.G.: Evaluation of esophageal tests in the diagnosis of reflux esophagitis. Gastroenterology *71:* 9–15 (1976).

89   Hillemeier, A.C.; Grill, B.B.; McCallum, R.; Gryboski, J.: Esophageal and gastric motor abnormalities in gastroesophageal reflux during infancy. Gastroenterology *84:* 741–746 (1983).

90   Benjamin, B.; Pohl, D.; Bale, P.M.: Endoscopy and biopsy and gastroesophageal reflux in infants and children. Ann. Otol. *89:* 443–445 (1980).

91   Biller, J.A.; Winter, H.S.; Grand, R.J.; Allred, E.N.: Are endoscopic changes predictive of histologic esophagitis in children? J. Pediat. *103:* 215–218 (1983).

92   Shub, M.D.; Ulshen, M.H.; Hargrove, C.B.; Siegal, G.P.; Groben, P.A.; Askin, F.B.: Esophagitis in infancy. A frequent consequence of gastroesophageal reflux. J. Pediat. *107:* 881–885 (1985).

93   Hargrove, D.B.; Ulshen, M.H.; Shub, M.D.: Upper gastrointestinal endoscopy in infants. Diagnostic usefulness and safety. Pediatrics, Springfield *74:* 828–831 (1984).

94   Kobayashi, S.; Kasugai, T.: Endoscopic and biopsy criteria for the diagnosis of esophagitis with a fiberoptic esophagoscope. Dig. Dis. *19:* 345–352 (1974).

95   Hogan, W.: Endoscopic diagnosis of esophageal disease. Pract. Gastroent. *1:* 17 (1979).

96   Behar, J.; Sheahan, D.C.: Histologic abnormalities in reflux esophagitis. Archs Path. *99:* 387–391 (1975).

97   Ismail-Beigi, F.; Horton, P.F.; Pope, C.E.: Histologic consequences of gastroesophageal reflux in man. Gastroenterology *58:* 163–174 (1970).

98   Johnson, L.F.; DeMeester, T.R.; Haggitt, R.C.: Esophageal epithelial response to gastroesophageal reflux. A quantitative study. Dig. Dis. *23:* 498–509 (1978).

99   Mitros, F.A.: Inflammatory and neoplastic diseases of the esophagus; in Appelman, Pathology of the esophagus, stomach and duodenum, pp. 1–35 (Churchill Livingstone, New York 1984).

100 Seefeld, U.; Krejs, G.J.; Siebenmann, R.E.; Blum, A.L.: Esophageal histology in gastroesophageal reflux. Dig. Dis. *22:* 956–964 (1977).

101 Weinstein, W.M.; Bogoch, E.R.; Bowes, K.L.: The normal human esophageal mucosa. A histological reappraisal. Gastroenterology *68:* 40–44 (1975).

102 Geboes, K.; Desmet, V.; Vantrappen, G.: Esophageal histology in the early stage of gastroesophageal reflux. Archs Pathol. Lab. Med. *103:* 205 (1979).

103 Geboes, K.; Desmet, V.; Vantrappen, G.; Mebis, J.: Vascular changes in the esophageal mucosa. Gastrointest. Endosc. *26:* 29–32 (1980).

104 Geboes, K.; DeWolf-Peeters, C.; Rutgeerts, P.; Janssens, J.; Vantrappen, G.; Desmet, V.: Lymphocytes and Langerhans' cells in the human oesophageal epithelium. Virchows Arch. Abt. A Path. Anat. *401:* 45–55 (1983).

105 Leape, L.L.; Lucian, L.; Bhan, I.; Ramenofsky, M.L.: Esophageal biopsy in the diag-
     nosis of reflux esophagitis. J. pediat. Surg. *16:* 379–384 (1981).

106 Pope, C.E.: Mucosal response to esophageal motor disorders. Archs intern. Med. *136:*
     549–555 (1976).

107 Brown, L.F.; Goldman, H.; Antonioli, D.A.: Intraepithelial eosinophils in endoscopic
     biopsies of adults with reflux esophagitis. Am. J. surg. Path. *8:* 899–905 (1984).

108 Mossberg, S.M.: The columnar-lined esophagus (Barrett syndrome). An acquired con-
     dition. Gastroenterology *50:* 671–676 (1966).

109 Naef, A.P.; Sovary, M.; Ozzello, L.: Columnar-lined lower esophagus. An acquired le-
     sion with malignant predisposition. Report on 140 cases of Barrett's esophagus with 12
     adenocarcinomas. J. thorac. cardiovasc. Surg. *70:* 826–834 (1975).

110 Dahms, B.; Rothstein, F.C.: Barrett's esophagus in children. A consequence of chronic
     gastroesophageal reflux. Gastroenterology *86:* 318–323 (1984).

111 Paull, A.; Trier, J.S.; Dalton, M.D.; Camp, R.C.; Loeb, P.; Goyal, R.K.: The his-
     tologic spectrum of Barrett's esophagus. New Engl. J. Med. *295:* 476–480 (1976).

112 Meyers, W.F.; Herbst, J.J.: Effectiveness of positioning therapy for gastroesophageal
     reflux. Pediatrics, Springfield *69:* 768–772 (1982).

113 Ramenofsky, M.L.; Leape, L.L.: Continuous upper esophageal pH monitoring in in-
     fants and children with gastroesophageal reflux, pneumonia, and apenic spells. J.
     pediat. Surg. *16:* 374–378 (1981).

114 Orenstein, S.R.; Whitington, P.F.: Positioning for prevention of infant gastro-
     esophageal reflux. J. Pediat. *103:* 534–537 (1983).

115 Euler, A.R.: Use of bethenechol for the treatment of gastroesophageal reflux. J.
     Pediat. *96:* 321–324 (1980).

116 Strickland, A.D.; Chang, J.H.: Results of treatment of gastroesophageal reflux with
     bethenechol. J. Pediat. *103:* 311–315 (1983).

117 Soundheimer, J.M.; Mintz, H.L.; Michaels, M.: Bethenechol treatment of gas-
     troesophageal reflux in infants. Effect on continuous esophageal pH records. J. Pediat.
     104: 128–131 (1984).

118 Behar, J.; Biancani, P.: Effect of oral metoclopramide on gastroesophageal reflux in
     the post-cibal state. Gastroenterology *70:* 331–335 (1976).

119 McCallum, R.W.; Ippoliti, A.F.; Cooney, C.; Sturdivant, A.L.: A controlled trial of
     metoclopramide in symptomatic gastroesophageal reflux. New Engl. J. Med. *296:* 354–
     357 (1977).

120 Stanciu, C.; Bennett, J.R.: Metoclopramide in gastroesophageal reflux. Gut *14:* 275–
     279 (1973).

121 Follette, D.; Fonkalsrud, E.W.; Euler, A.; Ament, M.: Gastroesophageal fundoplica-
     tion for reflux in infants and children. J. pediat. Surg. *76:* 757–764 (1976).

122 Schatzlein, M.H.; Ballentine, T.V.; Thirunavukkarasu, S.; Fitzgerald, J.F.; Grosfeld,
     J.L.: Gastroesophageal reflux in infants and children. Diagnosis and management.
     Archs Surg. *114:* 505–510 (1979).

123 Foglia, R.P.; Fonkalsrud, E.W.; Ament, M.E.; Byrne, W.J.; Berquist, W.; Siegel,
     S.C.; Katz, R.M.; Rachelefsky, G.S.: Gastroesophageal fundoplication for the man-
     agement of chronic pulmonary disease in children. Am. J. Surg. *140:* 72–79 (1980).

124 Leape, L.L.; Ramenofsky, M.L.: Surgical treatment of gastroesophageal reflux in chil-
     dren. Results of Nissen's fundoplication in 100 children. Am. J. Dis. Child. *134:* 935–
     938 (1980).

125 Carson, J.A.; Tunell, W.P.; Smith, E.I.: Pediatric gastroesophageal reflux. Age-specific indications for operation. Am. J. Surg. *140:* 768–771 (1980).

126 Johnson, D.G.; Jolley, S.G.; Herbst, J.J.; Cordell, L.J.: Surgical selection of infants with gastroesophageal reflux. J. pediat. Surg. *16:* suppl., pp. 587–594 (1981).

127 Johnson, D.G.; Jolley, S.G.: Gastroesophageal reflux in infants and children. Recognition and treatment. Surg. Clins N. Am. *61:* 1101–1115 (1981).

128 ONeill, J.A., Jr.; Betts, J.; Siegler, M.M.; Schnaufer, L.; Bishop, H.C.; Templeton, J.M.: Surgical management of reflux strictures of the esophagus in childhood. Ann. Surg. *196:* 453–460 (1982).

129 Woodward, E.R.: Surgical treatment of gastroesophageal reflux and its complications. Wld J. Surg. *1:* 453–461 (1977).

130 Hicks, L.M.; Christie, D.L.; Hall, D.G.; Cahill, J.L.; Mansfield, P.B.; Stevenson, J.K.; Bill, A.H.: Surgical treatment of esophageal stricture secondary to gastro-esophageal reflux. J. pediat. Surg. *15:* 863–868 (1980).

131 Tunell, W.P.; Smith, E.I.; Carson, J.A.: Gastroesophageal reflux in childhood. The dilemma of surgical success. Ann. Surg. *197:* 560–565 (1983).

132 Ashcraft, K.W.; Holder, T.M.; Amoury, R.A.: Treatment of gastroesophageal reflux in children by Thal fundoplication. J. thorac. cardiovasc. Surg. *82:* 706–712 (1981).

133 Harnsberger, J.K.; Corey, J.J.; Johnson, D.G.; Herbst, J.J.: Long-term follow-up of surgery for gastroesophageal reflux in infants and children. J. Pediat. *102:* 505–508 (1983).

134 Berquist, W.E.; Fonkalsrud, E.W.; Ament, M.E.: Effectiveness of Nissen fundoplication for gastroesophageal reflux in children as measured by 24-hour intraesophageal pH monitoring. J. pediat. Surg. *16:* 872–875 (1981).

135 Jolley, S.G.; Herbst, J.J.; Johnson, D.G.; Matlak, M.E.; Book, L.S.; Pena, A.: Postcibal gastroesophageal reflux in children. J. pediat. Surg. *16:* 487–490 (1981).

136 Papp, J.P.: Determination of the lower esophageal sphincter pressure in patients having a Nissen or Belsey fundoplication. Am. J. Gastroent. *71:* 154–157 (1979).

G.P. Siegal, MD, PhD, Department of Pathology, Brinkhous-Bullitt Building, 228 H, University of North Carolina School of Medicine, Chapel Hill, NC 27514 (USA)

Perspect. pediatr. Pathol., vol. 11, pp. 152–174 (Karger, Basel 1987)

Normal Anatomy of the Myenteric Plexus of Infants and Children

Demonstration by Flat-Mount (Circuit Diagram) Preparations[1]

Theadis R. Wells, Benjamin H. Landing, Ilana Ariel,
Rosario Nadorra, Caroline Garcia

Departments of Pathology and Pediatrics, Children's Hospital of Los Angeles, and
University of Southern California School of Medicine, Los Angeles, Calif., USA

Introduction

The nervous network of the gastrointestinal tract consists of at least six interconnected networks of nerve cell clusters (ganglia) joined by nerve fiber bundles, arranged concentrically in the wall of the gastrointestinal tract [1]. The largest of these networks, the myenteric or Auerbach plexus (MEP), lies in the intermuscular septum between the circular and longitudinal muscle layers of the gastrointestinal tract. The circuit diagram of the human MEP is poorly appreciated in conventional microscopic sections, which are usually taken with radial orientation, vertical to the planes of the layers of the bowel wall. Although abnormalities in neuron number or distribution, or in cytologic or histochemical properties of MEP nerve cells, are known in a number of diseases, and are employed for diagnostic purposes in gastrointestinal tract biopsies, e.g. aganglionic megacolon, neuronal lipidoses, the difficulty of demonstration of the 'circuit diagram' of the MEP by such methods has prevented adequate consideration of the possible role of structural abnormalities of the MEP in many conditions

---

[1] Presented as a Poster Presentation at the meeting of the Pediatric Pathology Club, Atlanta, Ga., Feb. 26–27, 1983, and at the 17th International Congress of Pediatrics, Manila, Philippines, Nov. 7–12, 1983. [Wells, T.R.; Landing, B.H.; Ariel, I.; Garcia, C.: Normal and abnormal anatomy of the myenteric plexus as shown in flat-mount ('circuit diagram') preparations. Lab. Invest. *48:* 16 (1983)].

with disordered gastrointestinal tract function. Since the fundamental studies of Irwin [2], using the guinea pig, other investigators have used his and similar flat-mount techniques for the study of the myenteric plexus in the frog and dog [3], rat [4], guinea pig [5], cat [6–8], opossum [9, 10] and monkey [11], but published studies of the MEP in humans have nearly been limited to radial and tangential [12–14] sectioning techniques, since the thickness of the muscle layers in the human alimentary tract limits visualization of the MEP in full thickness preparations. Kondratjew [3, 15–18], in a distinguished series of studies, however, has presented material from adults similar to that of this study, utilizing a more laborious method of block-staining with toluidine blue, clearing of the tissues with glycerin, and compressing the specimens between glass slides for optical-section photomicrography.

This paper describes a maceration-microdissection technique applicable to demonstration of the circuit diagram of the human MEP (the Auerbach layer) in relatively large specimens of gastrointestinal tract, and presents selected aspects of the normal anatomy of the MEP at various levels of the tract.

Methods

Maceration

Segments of alimentary tract are placed mucosal surface up on thick filter paper mounts, and fixed in 10% formalin for at least 7 days. Full thickness squares, 1 cm or larger in dimension, are transferred to small specimen jars, concentrated hydrochloric acid (15–20 ml) is added, and the jars are covered securely. Each jar is then placed in a standard staining dish containing 175–200 ml of 2–4% aqueous sodium bicarbonate solution (can be made with warm tap water, 45–50°C), and a smaller staining dish is inverted over the specimen jar, so that the level of the bicarbonate solution is about half the height of the jar, thereby creating an alkali trap to prevent escape of acid fumes. This apparatus is then placed in an incubator at 50–55°C for maceration, which takes approximately 1.5 h [19].

The degree of maceration should be checked every 20 min by gently rocking or swirling the jar containing the tissue. As maceration nears completion, the macerating fluid becomes brownish, the tissue takes on an undulating appearance and the mucosal layer may partially separate. After maceration, the cap of the tissue-containing jar is loosened beneath the surface of a tap-water-filled dish, which permits dilution of the acid, lowers the temperature of the fluid and prevents escape of fumes. The tissue is washed, either by holding the jar containing the tissue under a slow stream of water or by carefully removing the diluted acid with a syringe or dropper and replacing it with tap water 4 or 5 times. It is important that the bicarbonate solution not be allowed to contact the tissue at any time during maceration or washing.

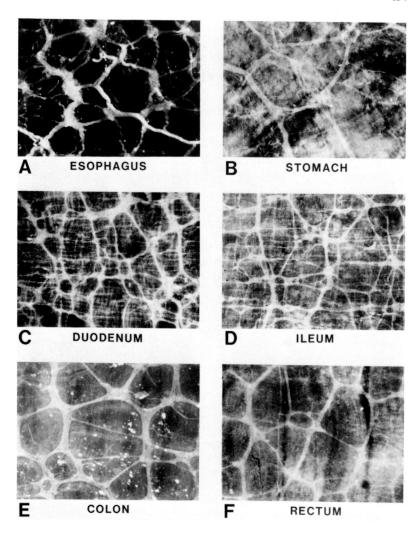

Fig. 1. Preparations of Auerbach plexus of esophagus, stomach, duodenum, ileum, colon and rectum. The mucosa and inner (circular) muscle layer have been removed for *B, C, D, E* and *F,* and both inner and external (longitudinal) muscle layers removed for *A. A* 5-8/12-year-old male with Down's syndrome. *B* 5-year-old male with Hurler's disease. *C* 12-year-old female with acute monocytic leukemia. *D* 8-9/12-year-old male with acute lymphatic leukemia. *E* Colon of same patient as in *(D). F* 14-year-old female with malignant lymphoma. ×20 reduced to ×16.

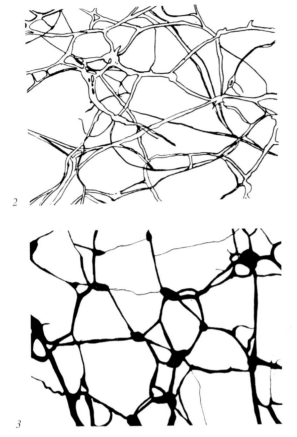

2

3

Fig. 2. Tracing of preparation of Auerbach plexus of stomach of 9-month-old female with Down's syndrome, showing the more complicated three-dimensional arrangement of this plexus in the stomach than in other regions of the gastrointestinal tract (cf. fig. 1, 3–13). ×20.

Fig. 3. Tracing of Auerbach layer preparation of upper esophagus of same patient as in figure 2, showing the relatively large, rounded, sharply outlined ganglia typical of the plexus in this region. ×20.

The proper degree of maceration can be determined by transferring the tissue into a Petri dish filled with distilled water, and teasing it with dissecting needles. If the tissue is hard, and separation of the layers is difficult, maceration can be repeated for an additional period. Adequately macerated tissue can be refrigerated for a week or longer in distilled water before dissection.

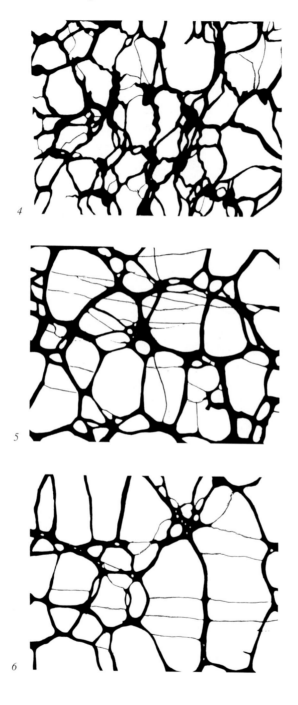

4

5

6

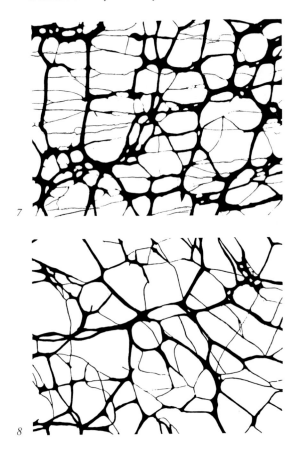

7

8

Fig. 4. Tracing of Auerbach plexus of mid-esophagus of same patient as in figures 2 and 3, showing greater fraction of neural tissue in the plane of the plexus than in the upper esophagus (fig. 2). ×20.

Fig. 5. Tracings of preparations of Auerbach plexus of duodenum, of same patient as in figures 2–4, showing greater fraction of neural tissue than in more distal small intestine. ×20.

Fig. 6. Tracing of jejunal Auerbach plexus from same patient as in figures 2–5, showing distinctive 'loose' widely-spaced network. ×20.

Fig. 7. Auerbach plexus of ileum of same patient as in figures 2–6, showing higher ratio of neural tissue (ganglia plus nerve trunks) than that of the jejunum (fig. 6). ×20.

Fig. 8. Tracing of preparation of Auerbach plexus of cecum of same patient as in figures 2–7, showing pattern similar to, but finer (with more slender nerve trunks) than that of the ileum (fig. 7). ×20.

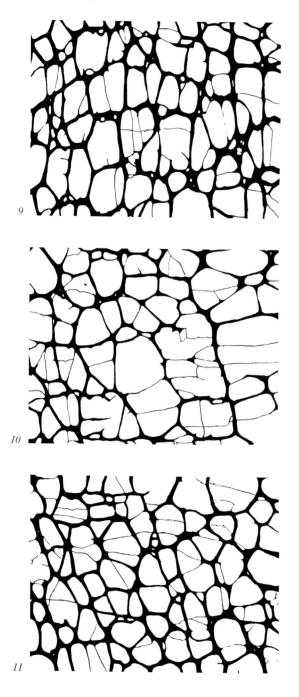

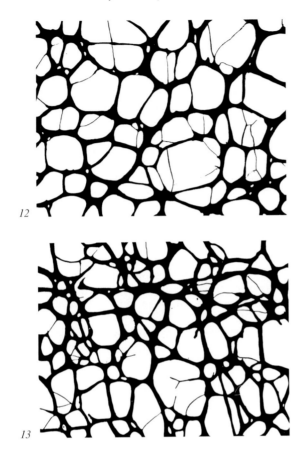

12

13

Fig. 9. Tracing of Auerbach plexus of ascending colon of same patient as in figures 2–8, showing denser network, with thicker nerve trunks than in the cecum. ×20.

Fig. 10. Tracing of transverse colon of same patient as in figures 2–9. ×20.

Fig. 11. Tracing of preparation of Auerbach plexus of descending colon of same patient as in figures 2–10. ×20.

Fig. 12. Tracing of Auerbach plexus of sigmoid colon of same patient as in figures 2–11, showing increasing thickness of nerve trunks in the more distal colon. ×20.

Fig. 13. Auerbach plexus of rectum of same patient as in figures 2–12, showing high 'relative fraction' of neural tissue in the plexus in this region, compared to that of the more proximal colon (fig. 8–12). ×20.

Dissection

Dissection is done with No. 11 or No. 16 beading needles (obtainable at handicraft stores) attached to paintbrush handles (water color type) with adhesive or cellophane tape.

Proper lighting of the specimens for dissection and photography is important, since light directed relatively vertically on the tissue can obscure the image by reducing contrast. The use of a black background is helpful, and light directed at about 45° to the specimen normally gives satisfactory contrast, although the best angle will vary considerably from specimen to specimen.

With the specimen placed mucosal surface down, one of the needles is placed in the submucosa, and the two muscular layers are separated from the submucosa and mucosa by the other needle. The muscle layers are then placed longitudinal (external) layer down, and the circular (inner) layer is removed by carefully removing small strips with the needles, leaving Auerbach's plexus visible on the inner surface of the longitudinal muscle layer (fig. 1). If the specimen begins to curl, small pieces of staples can be placed on the edges of the specimen. Because the MEP is more compact along the mesenteric border [20], the preparations illustrated in this study were taken along the antimesenteric border. Dissection of the gastric MEP is difficult because of its complicated three-dimensional arrangement, in contrast to the more two-dimensional Auerbach layer of the esophagus and of the small and large intestines (fig. 2). The exposed plexus can be photographed and/or drawn with a camera lucida. The preparations of this study were photographed with a Polaroid camera attached to a Wild M-7 stereomicroscope, using Type 665 positive/negative film (3¼ by 4¼). Tracings of transilluminated negatives, the negatives themselves, or the positive prints were utilized for the morphometric studies (fig. 2–13). The total magnification of these preparations is 20×. After photography, the specimens can be stored in 10% formalin for an indefinite period.

Morphometric Analysis

Morphometric analysis was performed, using a point count method [12], on preparations of 14 levels of the alimentary tract of a 9-month-old Caucasian female with Down's syndrome, who showed no clinical or pathologic evidence of gastrointestinal tract disease or abnormality. Each image was overlaid with a transparent grid having 165 test points. Hits on neural tissue (ganglia and nerve trunks) were recorded and divided by the total number of test points per field, giving relative fractions of plexus tissue to non-neural tissue. Comparable analysis was done on the drawings of the different levels of the guinea pig Auerbach plexus published by Irwin [2], using a larger grid with 225 test points because of the difference in dimensions of Irwin's figures compared to those in this paper (table I). Similar point-count analyses were done on 152 specimens of various levels of the gastrointestinal tract from 59 patients with no primary gastrointestinal disease, to establish the normative values (table II; fig. 17, 18). Analysis of these data gives the relation of the relative fraction of neural tissue in the Auerbach layers of different regions of the gastrointestinal tract in relation to age and body length through infancy and childhood (table III; fig. 14–18). The values for the patient whose specimens are illustrated in figures 1A and 2–14 fell within the normal ranges.

Data for comparison of the size of the MEP network at a given level of the gastrointestinal tract at different ages, and hence for calculation of the degree and rate of growth of the tract over various age periods, were also obtained by overlaying MEP tracings by a transparent sheet containing narrow parallel lines spaced 10 mm apart. The number of intersects of either ganglia or fiber bundles with these lines was counted for each preparation, and the ratios of these totals were calculated (table I; fig. 18).

Table I. Point-count and linear intersect analysis data

Gastrointestinal tract level	Point-count analysis		Irwin data point-count analysis		linear intersect analysis		
	average point-count	fraction neural tissue	average point-count	fraction neural tissue	mean number of intersects		±SD
Mid-esophagus	34.5/165 =	20%			6.2	±	1.5
Lower esophagus	50/165 =	30%	30/225 =	13%	7.7	±	2.6
Stomach	49/165 =	30%			10.1	±	2.5
Pylorus (at duodenum)	76.5/165 =	46%	78/225 =	35%	8.7	±	2.0
Duodenum, first portion	49/165 =	30%	57/225 =	25%	9.4	±	2.2
Duodenum, second portion	29/165 =	29%			10.4	±	1.5
Jejunum	27/165 =	16%			6.0	±	1.7
Ileum	48/165 =	29%	54/225 =	24%	13.7	±	2.3
Cecum	23.5/165 =	24%			10.0	±	1.8
Ascending colon	47/165 =	28%	69/225 =	31%	7.5	±	2.0
Transverse colon	47/165 =	28%			10.1	±	1.7
Descending colon	57/165 =	34%			9.6	±	1.5
Sigmoid colon	52.5/165 =	31%			7.5	±	1.4
Rectum	63.5/165 =	38%	50/225 =	22%	9.3	±	2.4
	Mean =	29.5%	mean =	25%	9.0	±	1.98

Data showing: (a) relative fraction of neural tissue in Auerbach layer of various regions of gastrointestinal tract of 9-month-old female with Down's syndrome (point count values give average of values obtained by analysis of the same preparations by two observers); (b) relative fraction of neural tissue in Auerbach layer of various regions of gastrointestinal tract of the guinea pig, based on figures given by Irwin [2], showing general parallelism of relative values for these two species; (c) values obtained by analysis of the same preparations as in (a) by counting the number of intersects of the network of the Auerbach plexus with a transverse line across the preparation. Values given are the mean number of intersects for ten traverses.

Results

Circuit diagrams were prepared of the Auerbach layer of the MEP of normal esophagus, stomach, duodenum, jejunum, ileum, cecum, colon (ascending, transverse, descending and sigmoid colon) and rectum of infants and children (fig. 1–13).

Table II. Relative fraction of neural tissue in the Auerbach plexus of various levels of the gastrointestinal tract of infants and children by body length

Height, cm	Esophagus	Stomach	Duodenum	Jejunum	Ileum	Cecum	Appendix	Colon	Rectum
50–85	0.29±0.06 (n=7)	0.22±0.07 (n=6)	0.31±0.10 (n=5)	0.25±0.04 (n=5)	0.34±0.05 (n=6)	0.32±0.04 (n=4)	0.28±0.07 (n=2)	0.32±0.06 (n=10)	0.33±0.07 (n=4)
86–121	0.25±0.05 (n=5)	0.23±0.06 (n=6)	0.27±0.03 (n=4)	0.27±0.04 (n=5)	0.27±0.07 (n=6)	0.20±0.03 (n=3)	0.24±0.06 (n=3)	0.28±0.07 (n=5)	0.39 (n=1)
122–157	0.35±0.08 (n=2)	0.23±0.08 (n=3)	0.34±0.04 (n=5)	0.20±0.02 (n=9)	0.21±0.04 (n=6)	0.18±0.06 (n=3)	0.18±0.01 (n=2)	0.19±0.03 (n=8)	0.25±0.04 (n=2)
158–193	0.19 (n=1)	0.21±0.05 (n=3)	0.28±0.04 (n=3)	0.18±0.04 (n=7)	0.19±0.04 (n=5)	0.18±0.02 (n=3)	0.14±0.01 (n=2)	0.19±0.02 (n=5)	0.21 (n=1)

Relative fraction of neural tissue in Auerbach plexus of various levels of the gastrointestinal tract of infants and children by body length, by the point-count technique, showing that the fraction falls and the network becomes coarser as the plexus 'stretches' with growth of the intestine for all regions of the GI tract from jejunum through colon, but changes less with age in esophagus, stomach, duodenum and rectum.

Table III. Analysis of relation of fraction of neural tissue in plane of Auerbach plexus at various levels of the small and large intestine to age and height

	n	Mean age months	Mean height cm	Mean fraction neural tissue	SD	Correlation coefficient		Probability	
						age	height	age	height
Esophagus	15	74.83	96.80	0.27	0.07	−0.10	−0.12	ns	ns
Stomach	18	90.11	107.75	0.22	0.06	−0.10	−0.04	ns	ns
Duodenum	17	106.77	112.59	0.30	0.07	−0.11	−0.08	ns	ns
Jejunum	26	133.26	127.60	0.22	0.05	−0.51	−0.60	<0.01	<0.01
Ileum	23	116.56	119.56	0.25	0.08	−0.69	−0.80	<0.001	<0.001
Cecum	13	123.73	115.96	0.23	0.07	−0.46	−0.72	ns	<0.01
Appendix	9	130.88	119.61	0.21	0.07	−0.65	−0.77	ns	<0.02
Colon	28	105.44	113.91	0.25	0.08	−0.80	−0.87	<0.001	<0.001
Rectum	8	70.00	99.81	0.30	0.08	−0.57	−0.59	ns	ns

Analysis of relation of fraction of neural tissue in plane of Auerbach plexus at various levels of the small and large intestine for age and height. The correlation coefficients for the relation between the fraction of neural tissue and the heights and body weights of the patients, analyzed for each locus, show better relation (the coefficient has a negative sign because the fractional value falls as the plexus stretches with growth) with body height than with weight. The growth of the MEP network thus appears to keep pace with body surface area rather than with body mass.

The general architecture of the Auerbach plexus (MEP) is a network of ganglia and interganglionic fiber bundles, with the spaces between the units of the meshwork of varying size and shape, throughout the alimentary tract [20]. With the exception of the gastric MEP, this plexus has a two-dimensional array of irregular polygons, but in the gastric MEP the polygons of the network have a three-dimensional array (fig. 2).

Some ganglia are separate structures, with well-defined boundaries, connected by varying numbers and sizes of interganglionic fibers. We use the term 'ganglionic complexes' for less sharply outlined structures lacking a sharp distinction between a single ganglion and two or more (fig. 1C, E) [21]. Because of these basic shapes of ganglia, we did not count the number of ganglia per unit area of plexus for computation of growth rates, but used values for neural tissue percentages per unit area. Generally, the interganglionic fiber connections appeared the same for the two types of ganglionic structures.

Esophagus

The esophageal MEP has a distinctive shape of the ganglia, which are predominantly solitary, ovoid and sharply distinguished from interganglionic fiber bundles (fig. 3, 4). The size and frequency of ganglia increase in the lower esophagus. The fiber bundles in the esophageal plexus appear rounder than do those at other levels of the gastrointestinal tract.

Stomach

The ganglia of the gastric MEP are smaller than those of the esophagus, and the interganglionic fiber trunks are relatively longer (fig. 1B). These structures have a three-dimensional [22] complex array of irregular polygons distributed over at least two levels, basically following the basket-woven architecture of the gastric muscularis. The most frequent forms of these polygons are pentagons and hexagons.

The pyloric ganglia have the same shape as those at other loci in the gastric plexus, but are larger, closer together, and with thicker interganglionic fiber bundles.

Duodenum

The coarser pattern of the plexus in the pylorus contrasts sharply with the finer pattern of the duodenum, and the proportion of neural tissue in the plane of the Auerbach plexus decreases from pylorus to duodenum to jejunum (fig. 5, 6).

Fig. 14. Fraction of the plane of the Auerbach plexus of various levels of gastrointestinal (GI) tract of 9-month-old female with Down syndrome, with no GI tract disease or abnormality, made up of neural tissue, established by point-count (solid line), compared to the relative fraction of neural tissue in the Auerbach layer of guinea pig GI tract at various loci determined by point-count analysis of the figures published by Irwin [2]. The general similarity of the relative amounts of neural tissue in the plane of the Auerbach plexus in different regions of the GI tract in the two species is apparent.

Fig. 15. Graph of relative fraction of neural tissue in the plane of the Auerbach plexus of the ileums of 23 patients ranging in age from the neonatal period to adolescence, showing that the fraction of neural tissue falls with age as the plexus 'stretches' with growth of the intestine.

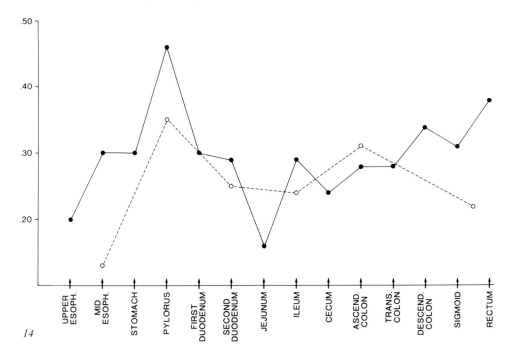

14

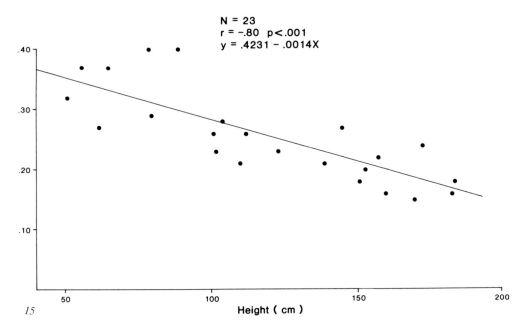

N = 23
r = −.80 p<.001
y = .4231 − .0014X

15

Height (cm)

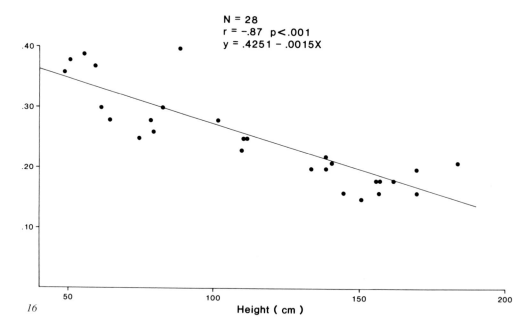

N = 28
r = −.87 p<.001
y = .4251 − .0015X

16

Height (cm)

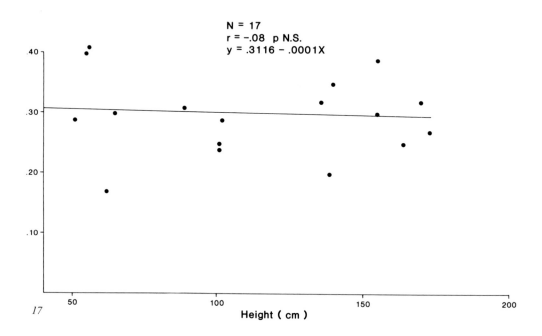

N = 17
r = −.08 p N.S.
y = .3116 − .0001X

17

Height (cm)

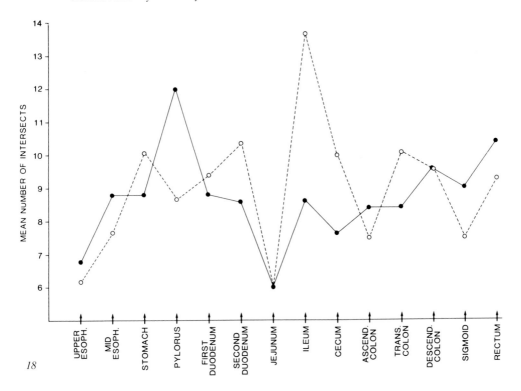

MEAN NUMBER OF INTERSECTS

UPPER ESOPH. MID ESOPH. STOMACH PYLORUS FIRST DUODENUM SECOND DUODENUM JEJUNUM ILEUM CECUM ASCEND COLON TRANS. COLON DESCEND. COLON SIGMOID RECTUM

18

Fig. 16. Graph of relative fraction of neural tissue in the plane of the Auerbach plexus of the colon of 28 patients ranging in age from the neonatal period to adolescence, showing that the fraction falls as the plexus 'stretches' with growth.

Fig. 17. Graph of relative fraction of neural tissue in the plane of the Auerbach plexus of the duodenum of 17 patients of varying ages and body lengths, from early infancy to adolescence, showing the relative lack of 'stretch' of the plexus with growth of the GI tract, suggesting that the length and circumference of this region of the GI tract increase less with age and body growth than do those of other regions of the small and large intestines (fig. 15, 16). Graph of point-count data for the stomachs of 18 patients over the same range of ages is similar to that for duodenum.

Fig. 18. Comparison of relative amounts of neural tissue in the Auerbach plexus (solid line: same data as in fig. 14) and the mean number of intersects of a transverse linear grid with the plexus in each of the preparations analyzed (dotted line: intersect data shown as vertical axis of graph). Differences between the two curves reflect primarily differences in thickness of interganglionic nerve trunks in the various regions of the GI tract. For example, the relatively high number of 'intersects' for ileum reflects the large number of very slender fibers in the ileal plexus (fig. 7). Similarly, the relatively low intersect count for pylorus, compared to the high fraction of neural tissue in the plane of the Auerbach plexus at this locus results from the high proportion of thick nerve trunks in this region.

Jejunum and Ileum

The MEP of the jejunum is distinctive because the widely spaced small ganglia and connecting fiber bundles form a looser network than is found at other levels (fig. 6). The network then gradually increases in relative fraction of neural components into the ileum. The pattern of the ileal MEP (fig. 7) is similar to that of the cecum (fig. 8), but the fiber trunks between the ganglia are more slender in cecum than in ileum. The ganglia in these regions, when solitary, are elongated and are usually aligned at right angles to the longitudinal muscle layer.

Appendix

The appendiceal MEP has the same basic pattern as that of the cecum, but with smaller ganglia and interganglionic fibers, so that its plexus has the most delicate network of any level of the alimentary tract. Emery and Underwood [23] have shown by a different technique that plexus of appendiceal type extends in the cecum to a point between the ileocal value and the orifice of the appendix.

Colon

The MEP through the ascending, transverse, descending and sigmoid colons is similar in pattern (fig. 9–12). The interganglionic fiber bundles are shorter and thicker than those of the small intestine, and the ganglia increase in size and number distally. The relative fraction of neural tissue in the descending colon is approximately 1.5 times that in the ascending and transverse colons. The plexus beneath the taeniae coli is more dense than it is in regions between taeniae [2, 5, 11, 13, 20, 21]. (The preparations of colon illustrated are from regions between taeniae.)

Rectum

The MEP of the rectum differs from that of the more proximal colon in increased size and frequency of ganglia and increased thickness of interganglionic fibers (fig. 13).

The point count data of this study (table I) were compared to data derived from point count analysis of the preparations illustrated in Irwin's [2] study of the myenteric plexus of the guinea pig. These curves (fig. 14) are very similar, and generally coincide with those given for numbers of ganglion cell in different regions of the gastrointestinal tract by Irwin [2]. Although absolute ganglion cell counts at the same levels of the tract differ for different species, the relative proportions of neural tissue and ganglion cell counts follow the same general course along the alimentary tract of the various species [21].

Various regions of 166 specimens of the gastrointestinal tract of 60 patients were analyzed as regards the relation between relative fraction of neural tissue in the Auerbach plexus layer, and the age and body length of the patients (table III). The data show generally better relation between the fraction of neural tissue in the Auerbach layer with height than with postnatal age, suggesting that growth in size of the small and large intestines is more related to body surface area (and to caloric need and nutrient demand) than to body mass.

Discussion

The normal circuit diagram anatomy of the Auerbach plexus at various levels of the gastrointestinal tract, at various ages through infancy and childhood, provides the basis for studies directed at demonstration of structural abnormalities of the plexus in disorders with proven or possible functional abnormalities of the gastrointestinal tract, e.g. Ariel and Wells [24], have shown deficiency of ganglia and fibers by the method described in this paper in the esophageal and gastric MEP in Riley-Day syndrome.

The pattern of the MEP accomplishes effective delivery of neural signals to the smooth muscle, and presumably also blood vessels and mucosa, of the gastrointestinal tract, the differences in pattern at different levels reflecting either differences in the amount of muscle to be controlled at different levels, the pacing or patterning of the instruction needed at each level, or both. Differences in MEP pattern at different levels of the gastrointestinal tract may reflect differences in the biochemical induction or maturation control signals operating during the early development of the plexus. As suggested by Bonner [25], anatomic patterns 'are achieved by a system of chemical signals' and 'the greater the distance over which the signals operate, the cruder the pattern'. The structure of the plexus must permit change in both longitudinal and transverse dimensions during dilatation and contraction of the intestinal tract. A pattern, or plane filler array, which most closely describes the plexus (with the exception of the stomach) is that of quadrilateral Dirichlet domains (fig. 19). As described by Loeb [26], with Dirichlet domains as plane fillers, any location within a domain lies closer to that domains's center than to that of any other, and every point in the plane belongs to only one domain. Inherent in this

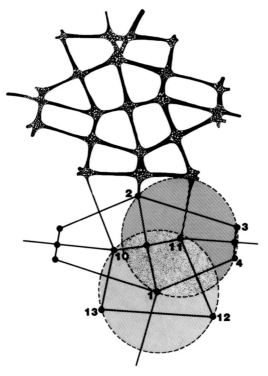

Fig. 19. The network of the Auerbach plexus can be considered as a set of polygonal areas outlined by nerve fiber trunks, with ganglia at the apices of the polygons. Any point within such a polygon (a Dirichlet domain) is closer to the center of that polygon than it is to the center of any other, and an apex is the same distance from the centers of all polygons any of the apical ganglia of which fall on a circle which has the specified ganglion at its center (e.g. ganglion No. 11 is the same distance from Nos. 1, 2, 3, 4, etc.). The arrangement imposes uniformity on nerve transmission distances (and times) between ganglionic neurons and smooth muscle fibers in different domains, and also explains the ability of the network to accomodate stretch in either direction as the intestinal tract distends or contracts.

arrangement is the ability to accommodate stretch in either direction. Its intrinsic network structure also gives the plexus the capacity to shunt electrical signals, in the event of local injury to ganglia and/or fracture of interganglionic fibers, around local defects in the network [27].

The MEP of the stomach, unlike the two-dimensional array of the esophagus and remaining gastrointestinal tract, is a three-dimensional geometric array. Minagawa et al. [22] have discussed the three-dimensional arrangement of the gastric MEP, but without specifying its precise pattern. This pattern resembles that of Dirichlet domains for a face-centered orthorhombic lattice, as described by Loeb [26].

Christensen provides quantitative data comparable to those of this study for the MEP of the opossum [9, 10], although muscularis stripping techniques, without some type of maceration, can cause disruption of segments of the plexus. We did not employ ganglion counts because of the occurrence of ganglionic complexes, in which what appear to be two, three or more ganglia are not easily separable one from another. As shown by Smith and Taylor [28], in the early development (65 mm crown-rump stage) of the myenteric plexus the neural tissue of the esophagus is a single fenestrated circumferential ganglion with irregular or relatively circular spaces. Patterson [29] has also shown that individual ganglia are not initially separate, but become so as growth progresses, perhaps explaining the ganglionic complexes.

Neuronal cell counts per unit area of bowel wall have a wide variation in neuron number at comparable loci of the gastrointestinal tract of different species, parallel to the great variation in the ratio of bowel length to body length for different species. Comparable variability can probably be expected for humans since, although the average ratio of bowel length/body length for humans is about 5:1 (range 3:1 – 6:1), this value can vary in different disease states from 1:1 to 10:1 [30].

The ratios of the relative fractions of neural tissue in the Auerbach layer of the duodenum and ileum derived by our pointcount method had a mean value of 1.3 (D/I=1.3), the same value found by Irwin [2] for the ratio of the number of nerve cells/cm^2 of guinea pig duodenum and ileum. It is of interest that the pace-setter potentials of the small intestine show a similar ratio of frequencies (humans; duodenum, 11/min; ileum, 8/min; D/I=1.4; dog; duodenum, 18/min; ileum, 13/min; D/I=1.4 [31].

Our technique for demonstration of the circuit-diagram of the Auerbach plexus of the gastrointestinal tract of young humans is applicable to study of the patterns of other levels, e.g. submucosal or Meissner plexus of the neural system of the tract. (An early demonstration of the human submucosal plexus is found in the first edition of Virchow's Cellularpathologie [32].) Abnormality of the pattern of the Auerbach plexus has been demonstrated in the esophagus and stomach of patients with Riley-Day syndrome (central autonomic dysfunction) [24], and quantitative abnormality (increase in relative fraction of neural tissue in the Auerbach layer) has been shown for ileum and colon in Crohn's disease and ulcerative colitis [33]. Analysis of qualitative and quantitative features of the Auerbach plexus in other neurologic and gastrointestinal disorders of infants and children will be of interest.

Conclusion

We present a method for demonstration and quantitation of the Auerbach layer of the human gastrointestinal tract in flat ('whole mount') preparations. The technique, which can be performed on fixed stored tissues, can be utilized for demonstration of both quantitive abnormalities and abnormalities in the pattern of the network of the plexus in various diseases. The structure of the plexus, which can, except for that of the stomach, be considered a plane-filling set of Dirichlet domains, explains its ability to accomodate change in dimension in either or both directions during dilatation and contraction. In the stomach the Auerbach plexus forms a three-dimensional array of ganglia and interganglionic fiber bundles.

The relative fraction of neural tissue (ganglia plus interganglionic fiber bundles) at all levels of the intestinal Auerbach plexus falls with age for jejunum, ileum, cecum, appendix and ascending, transverse and descending colons as the plexus 'stretches' with growth of the gastrointestinal tract. Present data do not establish whether this is also true for esophagus, stomach, duodenum and rectum. The relative fraction of neural tissue falls from duodenum to jejunum and rises again in the ileum. In the colon the fraction rises from ascending colon to rectum. The method provides a basis for studies of abnormalities of the pattern of the plexus in various diseases.

Acknowledgement

The authors are deeply indebted to Mrs. Peggy Earhart, who has again demonstrated her incomparable skill at preparation of manuscript.

Dedication

This paper is dedicated to the memory of Harley T. King, MS, of Tulsa, exceptional teacher of the principles of biological science, with gratitude for counsel and example.

References

1 Dupont, J.R.; Biggers, D.C.; Sprinz, H.: Intestinal renewal and immunosympathectomy. Archs Path. *80:* 357–362 (1965).

2 Irwin, D.A.: The anatomy of Auerbach's plexus. Am. J. Anat. *49:* 141–166 (1931).

3 Kondratjew, N.: Zur Frage nach der Nervengeflechte in der Bauchhöhle der Wirbeltiere. Z. Anat. *101:* 90–120 (1933).

4 Gabella, G.: Neuron size and number in the myenteric plexus of the newborn and adult rat. J. Anat. *109:* 81–95 (1971).

5 Matsuo, H.: A contribution on the anatomy of Auerbach's plexus. Jap. J. med. Sci. Anat. *4:* 417–428 (1934).

6 Stöhr, P., Jr.: Mikroskopische Studien zur Innervation des Magen-Darmkanales 1. Zs. Zellforsch. mikrosk. Anat. *12:* 67–154 (1931).

7 Leaming, D.B.; Canna, N.: A qualitative and quantitative study of the myenteric plexus of the small intestine of the cat. J. Anat. *95:* 160–169 (1961).

8 Richardson, K.C.: Studies on the structure of autonomic nerves in the small intestine, correlating the silver-impregnated image in light microscopy with the permanganate-fixed ultrastructure in electron microscopy. J. Anat. *94:* 457–472 (1960).

9 Christensen, J.; Robison, B.A.: Anatomy of the myenteric plexus of the opossum esophagus. Gastroenterology *83:* 1033–1042 (1982).

10 Christensen, J.; Rick, G.A.; Robison, B.A.; Stiles, M.J.; Wix, M.A.: Arrangement of the myenteric plexus throughout the gastrointestinal tract of the opossum. Gastroenterology *85:* 890–899 (1983).

11 Ohkubo, K.: Studien über das intramurale Nervensystem des Verdauungskanals. III. Affe und Mensch. Jap. J. med. Sci. Anat. *6:* 219–247 (1936).

12 Emery, J.L.; Finch, E.; Lister, J.: Use of circumferential tangential cryostat sections of the intestine in the diagnosis of Hirschsprung's disease. J. clin. Path. *20:* 263–266 (1967).

13 Smith, B.: The neuropathology of the alimentary tract (Williams & Wilkins, Baltimore 1972).

14 Lake, B.D.; Nixon, H.H.; Claireaux, A.E.: Hirschsprung's disease. Archs Pathol. Lab. Med. *102:* 244–247 (1978).

15 Kondratjew, N.: Zur Lehre von der Mageninnervation beim Menschen: 1. Mitt. Z. Anat. *86:* 320–347 (1928).

16 Kondratjew, N.: Zur Lehre von der Mageninnervation beim Menschen: 2. Mitt. Z. Anat. *89:* 328–343 (1929).

17 Kondratjew, N.: Zur Lehre von der Mageninnervation beim Menschen: 3. Mitt. Über die nervösen Wechselbeziehungen in der Gegend des Sphincter pylori beim Menschen. Z. Anat. *93:* 765–774 (1930).

18 Kondratjew, N.: Zur Lehre von der Innervation der Bauch- und Beckenhöhleorgane beim Menschen: 2. Mitt. Über intramural nervöse Wechselbeziehungen im Menschendarm. Z. Anat. *93:* 775–789 (1930).

19 Wells, T.R.: A rapid method of maceration for microdissection. Am. J. clin. Path. *47:* 349–350 (1967).

20 Gabella, G.: Structure of the autonomic nervous system (Chapman & Hall, London 1976).

21 Gabella, G.: Innervation of the gastrointestinal tract. Int. Rev. Cytol. *59:* 129–193 (1979).

22 Minagawa, H.; Shiosaka, S.; Inoue, H.; Hayashi, N.; Kasahara, A.; Kamata, T.; To-
    hyama, M.; Shiotani, Y.: Origins and three-dimensional distribution of substance P-
    containing structures on the rat stomach using whole-mount tissue. Gastroenterology
    86: 51–59 (1984).

23 Emery, J.L.; Underwood, J.: The neurological junction between the appendix and the
    ascending colon. Gut 11: 118–120 (1970).

24 Ariel, I.; Wells, T.R.: Structural abnormalities of the myenteric (Auerbach) plexus in
    familial dysautonomia (Riley-Day syndrome), as demonstrated by flat mount prepara-
    tion of the esophagus and stomach. Pediat. Path. 4: 89–98 (1985).

25 Bonner, J.T.: On development (Harvard Press, Cambridge 1974).

26 Loeb, A.: Space structures. Their harmony and counterpoint (Addison-Wesley, Read-
    ing 1976).

27 Furness, J.B.; Costa, M.: Neurons with 5-hydroxytryptaminelike immunoreactivity in
    the enteric nervous system. Their projections in the guinea pig small intestine. Neuro-
    science 7: 341–349 (1982).

28 Smith, R.B.; Taylor, I.M.: Observations on the intrinsic innervation of the foetal
    oesophagus between the 10 mm and 140 mm crown-rump length stages. Acta Anat. 81:
    127–138 (1972).

29 Patterson, M.W.H.: The prenatal intrinsic innervation of the gastroesophageal region;
    thesis, University of Manchester, 1961 (Quoted by Smith and Taylor, [28]).

30 Reiquam, C.W.; Allen, R.P.; Akers, D.R.: Normal and abnormal small bowel lengths.
    Am. J. Dis. Child. 109: 447–451 (1965).

31 Szurszewski, J.H.: Why pace the pacesetter potential of the small intestine? Mayo Clin.
    Proc. 57: 530–531 (1982).

32 Virchow, R.: Die Cellularpathologie in ihrer Begründung auf physiologische und
    pathologische Gewebelehre, fig. 87, p. 228 (Berlin, 1858).

33 Nadorra, R.; Landing, B.H.; Wells, T.R.: The intestinal plexuses in Crohn's disease
    and ulcerative colitis in children: pathologic and microdissection studies. Pediat. Path.
    (in press).

B.H. Landing, MD, Anatomic Pathology Division,
Childrens Hospital of Los Angeles, 4650 Sunset Boulevard,
Los Angeles, CA 90027 (USA)

Perspect. pediatr. Pathol., vol. 11, pp. 175–192 (Karger, Basel 1987)

Indian Childhood Cirrhosis

Vijay V. Joshi

Department of Pathology, Children's Hospital of New Jersey, United Hospitals
Medical Center and University of Medicine and Dentistry of New Jersey, New Jersey
Medical School, Newark, N.J., USA

History

In the West, it is customary to look for descriptions of seemingly recent medical disorders in the writings of ancient Greek physicians, particularly Hippocrates. In India, it is customary to look to ancient Sanskrit literature on medical disorders. According to some Sanskrit medical scholars
in India, the Susruta Samhita (1000 BC) contains reference to a disorder
resembling Indian childhood cirrhosis (ICC) [1–3], although Sen [4] provided the first description of the disease in more recent Indian medical literature in 1887 and Radhakrishna Rao [5] described the pathologic findings in 1935. In 1955, the Liver Diseases Sub-Committee of the Indian
Council of Medical Research [6] produced a detailed review of ICC and
added their own findings to the current knowledge. From review of 50
cases of ICC studied at the University of Delhi, Smetana et al. [7]
suggested a nutritional basis to the pathogenesis. Some of the more recent
contributions to clinical, pathological, pathogenetic and epidemiological
aspects of ICC [8–14] have focussed on the vastly increased amounts of
copper in the liver [10–12].

Terminology and Definition

The term Indian childhood cirrhosis (ICC) describes the age and
geographic incidence without reference to etiopathogenesis (which has not

been established) and replaces previously used terms such as infantile cirrhosis of liver in India, subacute toxic cirrhosis of infants and biliary cirrhosis in children.

Whether the lesion represents a cirrhotic process has been questioned [7, 15, 16] due to the paucity of regenerative activity and vague nodularity of the liver parenchyma. The International Study Group [17] sponsored by WHO defines cirrhosis 'as a diffuse process characterized by fibrosis and conversion of normal liver architecture into structurally abnormal nodules' and does not require regenerative activity as a criterion.

Despite the need for a precise, specific definition of ICC [18, 19] no single unique clinical, pathologic or biochemical feature marks each case, leaving only a descriptive definition consisting of a set of clinicopathologic criteria.

The Liver Diseases Sub-Committee [6] of the Indian Council of Medical Research described ICC in 1955: 'Infantile cirrhosis of liver is a disease peculiar to India affecting infants and young children with a tendency to run in families. It is characterized in the early stages by enlargement of liver which is felt to be hard and usually also of spleen with ascites and jaundice superimposed in the later stages. Its onset is insidious with vague symptomatology, course variable but generally rather slow and termination usually fatal. Its etiology is unknown.'

Morphologic features of ICC include the two basic features of intralobular pericellular fibrosis and intracellular orcein-positive coarse granules and the additional features of hepatocellular degeneration and Mallory's hyaline [8, 19–22].

From a variety of sources we propose clinicopathologic guidelines for a working definition of ICC: a chronic liver disease of undetermined etiology peculiar to Indian infants and young children with several clinical and pathologic features: (a) insidious onset, vague gastrointestinal symptoms, hepatomegaly and tendency to familial incidence; (b) normal ceruloplasmin and elevated serum glutamic oxalacetic transferase values in the blood; (c) micronodular cirrhosis with poor nodule formation, continued hepatocellular injury, Mallory's hyaline, lack or paucity of regenerative activity, creeping intercellular fibrosis, intralobular and portal inflammatory infiltrate, increased orcein-staining copper-associated protein in the hepatocytes and absence of fatty change. Because of absence of diagnostic clinical features and discriminatory liver function tests, the pathologic features have paramount importance in the diagnosis of ICC.

Epidemiology

Although the precise incidence of ICC is not known, it accounts for more than half of the chronic liver diseases in children in India [14, 23]. ICC affects infants and young children between 4 months and 5 years; 75% of the patients are aged 1–3 years [8]. The markedly higher incidence in hospitalized boys (M:F ratio 4:1) may partly reflect the prevailing sociocultural factors favoring care for males. In field studies and other hospital surveys sex incidence is nearly equal [6, 9, 23].

Although initially reported from eastern India, ICC has subsequently been described from all parts of India and rarely from other parts of the world including western countries (vide infra). ICC occurs predominantly in children of the social middle class, affecting Hindus, including Jains and Sikhs, preferentially with a higher frequency in certain castes such as Brahmin, Agarwal and Kayastha [6, 8, 9].

Family Incidence: Based on a family history of liver disease and liver function test values and liver biopsy in siblings of affected children, 25–30% of cases of ICC are familial. Although a segregation ratio of 0.2196 by pedigree analysis is compatible with autosomal recessive inheritance [24], the data are inconclusive, suggesting a multifactorial origin with a strong genetic component (85%) [25].

Clinical Aspects

ICC has three clinical stages: early, intermediate and late [6, 26]. The early stage has an insidious onset characterized by disturbances of appetite and bowel movement, occasionally jaundice and slight enlargement of a firm liver with a sharp edge. The intermediate stage is characterized by irritability, minimal jaundice, marked hepatomegaly, leafy edge (i.e. a sharp thin edge like that of a leaf), splenomegaly and occasionally by subcutaneous edema, ascites and susceptibility to infection. The late stage is characterized by increased jaundice, hepatomegaly, splenomegaly, and terminal precoma or coma. Portal hypertension can occur in this stage but it is uncommon [7]. Terminally, ICC may progress to hepatocellular failure with hepatic coma. Intercurrent infection or gastrointestinal bleeding are occasional complications.

The clinical differential diagnosis of ICC includes other chronic liver diseases such as chronic active hepatitis and other forms of cirrhosis [27].

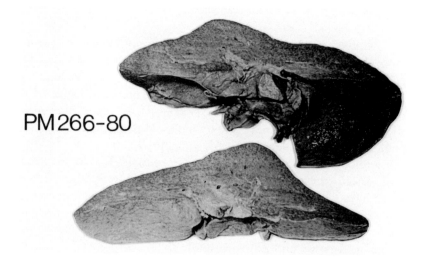

Fig. 1. The liver in ICC has a sharp edge and granular to finely nodular external surface (upper slice). Dark (green) fine nodules separated by white fibrous septa are seen on the cut surface of the lower slice.

Results of standard clinical laboratory tests reflect liver dysfunction in ICC [6, 8, 14] but do not discriminate from other chronic liver disorders of childhood.

Pathology

Histopathologic features in a liver biopsy constitute objective, definitive evidence of ICC. From the few descriptions of gross appearances of the liver [2, 18], the enlarged, firm liver has a granular to finely nodular external surface and leafy sharp edge. The cut surface has the small (0.5–2 mm) indistinct to distinct nodules (fig. 1) of micronodular cirrhosis. Rarely, the liver may have normal or slightly reduced size and large areas of fibrosis without discernible nodularity [2, 18, 28] (fig. 2).

Histologically the liver in ICC has several characteristic features: (a) continuing hepatocellular injury; (b) fibrosis, (c) paucity or absence of regenerative activity; (d) nodularity, and (e) inflammation.

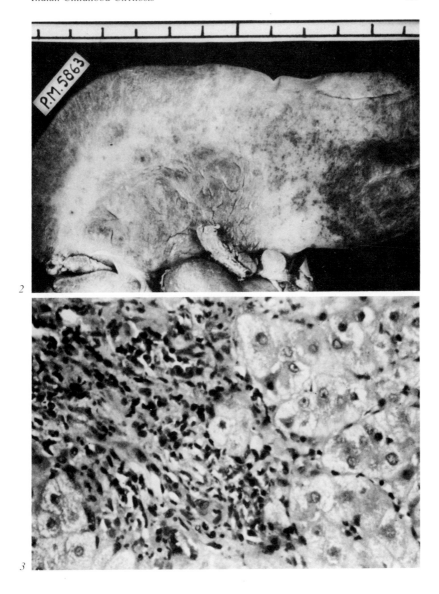

Fig. 2. The cut surface of liver in ICC has white streaks and large white fibrous areas.

Fig. 3. Histologically, the liver in ICC has ballooning of hepatocytes with rarefaction and clumping of the cytoplasm. The centrally located nucleolus in some of the hepatocytes presents a bird's eye appearance. Creeping fibrosis extends within the parenchyma with moderately dense inflammatory cell infiltrate in the fibrous tissue and the parenchyma. HE. ×250.

Continuing hepatocellular injury manifests as ballooned hepatocytes with rarefied clumped cytoplasmic contents and indistinct outline of the cell membrane. A centrally located nucleolus in a vesicular nucleus gives the nuclei a 'bird's eye' appearance [7] (fig. 3). Some hepatocytes appear necrotic as evidenced by clumped or homogeneous markedly eosinophilic cytoplasm, pyknotic or absent nucleus and loss of cellular outline. Mallory's hyaline (fig. 4) which, according to Nayak et al. [20], can be demonstrated in every case of ICC usually affects about 15% of the hepatocytes, but in rapidly progressive and fatal cases may affect the majority of hepatocytes. Despite the profound hepatocellular injury fatty change is characteristically absent [8].

Fibrosis characteristically occurs between small groups of hepatocytes in a pattern that has been described as creeping intercellular fibrosis (fig. 3, 5). Fatal cases may have large areas of fibrosis with only a few surviving hepatocytes.

Despite the extensive hepatocellular injury, regeneration as judged from the paucity of enlarged nuclei, binucleate hepatocytes and widening of hepatic cell plates, is minimal or absent.

Focal and indistinct micronodule formation (fig. 6) reflects the minimal regenerative activity and the predominantly intralobular, intercellular distribution of fibrosis.

A variable degree of inflammatory infiltrate consisting mostly of mononuclear cells and some neutrophils, is present within the parenchyma, portal tracts and fibrous septa (fig. 3) with satellitosis by neutrophils around degenerating or necrotic hepatocytes.

A variable degree of hepatocellular and canalicular cholestasis accompanies a constant ductular proliferation. Focally, the lobular and sublobular veins compressed by fibrous tissue have subendothelial sclerosis.

An increased amount of hepatocellular cytoplasmic copper and copper-associated protein is indicated by orcein and rhodanine posititive coarse granules [12, 31, 32] (fig. 7).

Electron microscopy [3, 12, 33, 34] confirms the degenerative changes in the hepatocytes and the diffusely scattered fibrosis. Hepatocytes contain electron-lucent cytoplasmic areas related to both a paucity and a loose arrangement of the organelles. Hepatocytes have dilated cisterns of rough endoplasmic reticulum, indistinct outlines of mitochondrial membrane and cristae, numerous lysosomes. Mallory's hyaline with its finely fibrillar structure and irregular dense bodies probably representing cuprosomes (fig. 8, 9).

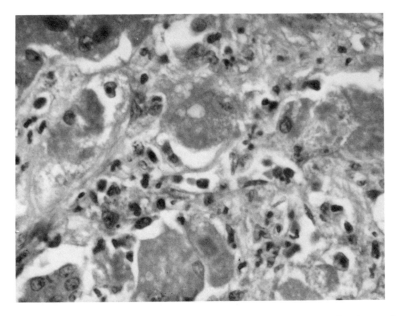

Fig. 4. Notable features of liver in ICC include Mallory's hyaline, occasional necrotic cell and inflammatory cell infiltrate. HE. ×400.

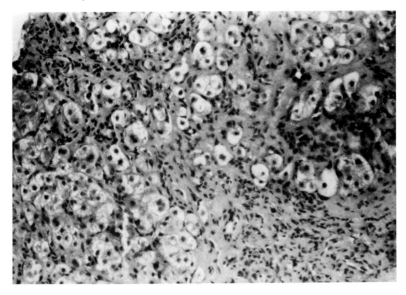

Fig. 5. The liver in ICC may have intralobular fibrosis between single or small clusters of cells, ballooning of hepatocytes, and only a vague suggestion of nodularity. HE. ×250.

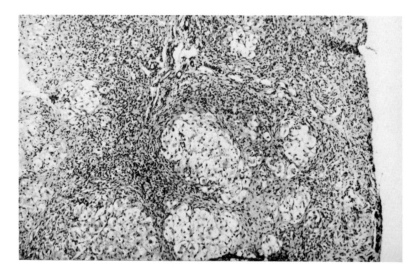

Fig. 6. Focally, the liver has fairly well-marked micronodules surrounded by fibrosis accentuating a few small clusters of cells and large areas of fibrosis. There is also ballooning of hepatocytes and an inflammatory cell infiltrate in the fibrous tissue. HE. ×100.

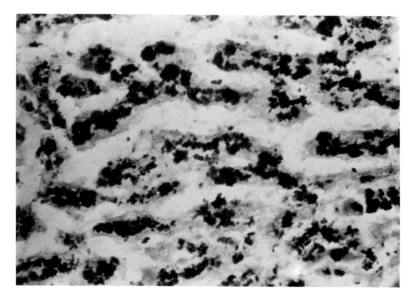

Fig. 7. The liver in ICC may have abundant coarse granular deposits. Orcein. ×250.

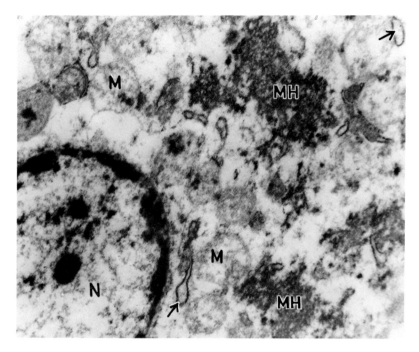

Fig. 8. Electron micrograph of a portion of hepatocytes from an autopsy specimen of ICC showing nucleus (N), Mallory's hyaline (MH), mitochondria with indistinct outlines (M) and dilated rough endoplasmic reticulum (arrows). Uranyl acetate and lead citrate. ×10,000. Courtesy: Dr. A.G. Bhagwat, Chandigarh, India.

Staging of Pathologic Features

Three stages or grades of progressive pathologic changes have been identified [7, 26]: (1) stage of injury – characterized by mild ballooning degeneration, Mallory's hyaline in occasional hepatocytes, portal fibrosis without cirrhosis; (2) stage of progressive degeneration and necrosis – cholestasis, inflammatory infiltrate and creeping fibrosis added to the features of stage of injury, and (3) evolution of cirrhosis – extensive fibrosis and Mallory's hyaline in over 75% of hepatocytes. The minimal regenerative activity, when present, is seen in this stage. These three stages of pathologic changes correlate with the clinical stages of early, intermediate and late.

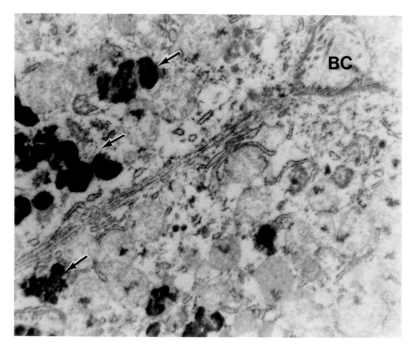

Fig. 9. Electron micrograph of portions of cytoplasm of two hepatocytes showing irregular dense bodies (arrows) probably representing cuprosomes. BC=Bile canaliculus. Uranyl acetate and lead citrate. ×4,500. Courtesy: Dr. A.G. Bhagwat, Chandigarh, India.

Etiopathogenesis

Despite extensive study, the precise etiopathogenesis of ICC remains undetermined. Several factors remain under consideration.

Viral hepatitis (A and B) does not appear to play a significant role in the pathogenesis of ICC [24, 31] since patients with ICC seldom have a history of contact with known cases of hepatitis; epidemics of hepatitis carry no increased incidence of ICC in the population at risk [35]; patients with ICC have absent or low hepatitis B surface antigenemia and liver cells have no surface or core components of hepatitis B virus as determined by immunoperoxidase, immunofluorescence, orcein staining and electron microscopy [31].

Serologically patients with ICC have a high frequency of hepatitis B, Epstein-Barr virus and cytomegalovirus infection but none have been specifically associated with ICC. Markers for other viruses such as non-A, non-B hepatitis have not been thoroughly studied.

Aflatoxin, a hepatotoxin produced by the rapidly growing fungus, *Aspergillus flavus,* commonly contaminates grain, peanuts and animal feed stored under warm and humid conditions in certain parts of India [37] and appears in milk of cows and buffalos. Aflatoxin B_1 has been identified in some cases of ICC but not in others [39]. Three children with Kwashiorkor who were fed peanut protein flour which had been contaminated with aflatoxin developed liver damage progressing from severe fatty change to fibrosis [40]. Although the hepatic lesion of aflatoxin-induced liver disease in experimental animals has some similarity to that in ICC, the aflatoxin-induced lesion has no Mallory's hyaline, the hallmark of ICC. Aflatoxin contamination occurs in many African and Asian countries. The geographic confinement of ICC to India fails to implicate aflatoxin in the etiopathogenesis of ICC.

Since both ICC and alcoholic liver disease are marked by Mallory's hyaline, Smetana et al. [7] suggested a nutritional role in ICC. However, ICC primarily affects children of middle-class families who do not have protein calorie malnutrition. Furthermore, the liver in ICC lacks the fatty change of nutritional liver disease.

Immunologic abnormalities which probably reflect hepatocellular damage and chronic debilitation in patients with ICC include hypergammaglobulinemia, reduced levels of B_1C complement component, reduced phytohemagglutinin induced blast cell transformation, depressed delayed hypersensitivity as measured by skin tests [24, 41, 42], thymic atrophy and reduced number of peripheral T cells [8, 26].

Patients with ICC have aminoaciduria [43] and large amounts of tryptophan metabolites, particularly 3-hydroxyanthranilic acid, in the urine [2] probably secondary to liver damage.

Kapoor et al. [44] attributed the hypercupremia accompanying ICC to liver cell necrosis, erythrocyte destruction, chronic infection and high levels of unmetabolized estrogens. Nayak et al. [31] illustrated the coarse orcein-positive hepatocytic granules believed to represent the sulfydryl-rich copper-binding proteins [32]. The liver in ICC has high levels of copper up to 4,788 μg/g with an average of 1,389$\pm$525 μg/g of dry liver tissue compared to the normal range of 15–55 μg/g [11, 12]. Although elevated hepatic copper content is found in neonatal livers and accompanies hepatic disorders such as Wilson's disease, primary biliary cirrhosis, cholestatic hepatitis and extrahepatic biliary obstruction, the copper concentration in

ICC reaches higher levels and a more diffuse intralobular distribution than in the other conditions [11, 32, 45, 46].

Excessive copper may alter the assembly of microtubules in the hepatocytes leading to the accumulation of intermediate filaments constituting the Mallory's hyaline and interfere with intracellular transport leading to retention of secretory protein and resultant ballooning of hepatocytes [12]. Brass and copper household utensils have been suggested as a possible source of copper exposure [21, 47]. Boiling and storing of milk in unplated metal utensils, a common practice in rural areas, raises its copper concentration from 11.5 ± 3.6 to 625 ± 2.4 $\mu g/100$ ml. Water takes up copper to a lesser extent. Furthermore the average age of introduction of top feeding of animal milk is significantly earlier in children with ICC (at mean age of 4.9 vs. 9.4 months in control children) – thus exposing them to high concentrations of copper at an early age [21].

It is not clear whether high hepatic copper concentration is due to a primary inherited metabolic defect peculiar to certain Indian children, is secondary to hepatic damage and cholestasis or is due to environmental exposure to high concentrations of copper. Copper homeostasis is maintained by intestinal absorption and biliary excretion as the two major factors with ceruloplasmin probably involved in the transport of copper from the liver to the other tissues. The liver is the main recipient of absorbed copper, the site of production of ceruloplasmin and the principal excretory organ for copper. Biliary excretion of copper tends to vary in response to copper intake. Biliary excretion is less responsive to copper intake in certain animals and these animals lack the capacity to manage copper homeostasis by altering copper excretion in the bile. This leads to high concentration of copper in the liver if there is excessive intake [48, 49].

Patients with Wilson's disease have reduced serum ceruloplasmin levels, reduced biliary excretion of copper and increased levels of copper in the liver and cultured fibroblasts. Patients with ICC have normal or raised serum ceruloplasmin levels [44] and apparently normal copper metabolism in the cultured fibroblasts [49, 50].

The hepatic copper content in the early stages of ICC and extent of biliary excretion of copper are not known. Histochemically, Marwaha and co-workers [51, 52] found moderately high amounts of hepatic copper in asymptomatic siblings of patients with ICC but quantitation in clearly defined early cases of the disease has not been performed.

ICC occurs in families but without a precise pattern of inheritance. Potential hereditary factors include abnormality of copper metabolism and persistance of fetal hepatocytes. Alphafetoprotein (AFP), a marker of fetal or immature hepatocytes normally present in the serum of neonates, normally disappears rapidly after birth and cannot be detected by gel diffusion technique within a few weeks after birth. Transformation from fetal to adult hepatocytes suppresses AFP synthesis [53, 54]. AFP was detected by gel-diffusion technique in sera of 45% of children with ICC, most of whom were over 1 year of age [55], suggesting persistence of fetal hepatocytes as a genetically determined abnormality. With this hypothesis, vulnerability of fetal hepatocytes to environmental toxins may initiate the pathologic process of ICC. However, high AFP levels persist in other hepatic diseases of infants and children [55].

Indications for a multifactorial pathogenesis of ICC include exposure to hepatotoxic environmental factors at a vulnerable age in a genetically predisposed child resulting in chronic liver disease, followed by inanition and immunologic deficiency which aggravate the vulnerability to the same or additional hepatotoxins. Environmental factors may include infectious agents such as hepatitis viruses and toxic agents such as aflatoxin and excessive copper.

Differential Diagnosis

Although ICC has no single pathognomonic feature, the combination of morphologic features is diagnostic excluding other types of cirrhosis with the possible exception of Wilson's disease. Differential diagnosis of ICC includes those conditions prevalent in India which share one or more clinicopathologic features with ICC and show a familial incidence.

Heredofamilial and Metabolic Cirrhosis

Wilson's disease, because of its familial incidence, occurrence in childhood, presence of Mallory's hyaline in the cirrhotic stage and increased amount of hepatic copper with copper-associated protein resembles ICC. Wilson's disease has a later onset than ICC, characteristic Kayser-Fleischer rings and hepatocellular fatty change. Mallory's hyaline is not as abundant in Wilson's disease as in ICC and the copper concentrates in selected nodules or distinct foci. Copper in ICC is present diffusely in all hepatocytes [12]. The cirrhosis in Wilson's disease is macronodular without creeping fibrosis.

Postinfectious and Toxic Cirrhoses

Congenital syphilis stimulates pericellular fibrosis in the liver resembling that seen in ICC but does not contain Mallory's hyaline and ICC lacks the stigmata of congenital syphilis. Cirrhosis following viral hepatitis has no specific histologic markers except for HBsAg in the hepatocytes which may be present in the patients who have cirrhosis due to other causes. Posthepatitic cirrhosis is usually macronodular and lacks Mallory's hyaline. Clinically, chronic active hepatitis may be misdiagnosed as ICC [14, 27] – but liver biopsy characteristically shows piecemeal necrosis and no Mallory's hyaline. Aflatoxin toxicity results in perivenous collagenosis, centrilobular scarring, syncytial transformation and ballooning degeneration of hepatocytes progressing to cirrhosis but no Mallory's hyaline [57, 58]. Chronic veno-occlusive disease which is endemic in Jamaica and has been reported from India [59] is probably caused by pyrolizidine alkaloids from Crotolaria and Senecio species. Macronodular cirrhosis with centrilobular fibrosis gives the appearance of 'reversed lobulation'. Subintimal fibrosis and thrombosis obliterates centrilobular or sublobular hepatic veins. Similar type of cirrhosis but without creeping fibrosis of the parenchyma and Mallory's hyaline is seen in Budd-Chiari syndrome associated with occlusion of large hepatic veins near their entrance into vena cava. Cirrhosis of undetermined etiology may have no well-defined pattern or may be macronodular but lacks the degenerative change and Mallory's hyaline of ICC.

Comment

Despite the availability of considerable data on ICC, the diagnosis of ICC lacks a consensus on definition and minimum criteria. In the absence of discriminatory clinical and biochemical markers, pathologic features in the liver assume major diagnostic importance.

Bhagwat et al. [3] propose 10 clinicopathologic criteria for the diagnosis of ICC: (1) age: 10–24 months; (2) firm, smooth hepatomegaly extending 3 cm or more below the costal margin; (3) sharp leafy edge of the liver; (4) splenomegaly; (5) serum glutamic oxalacetic transferase greater than 260 IU; (6) periportal to panlobular coarse, hepatocytic orcein-positive deposits; (7) Mallory's hyaline with satellitosis; (8) excess copper by qualitative (rubeanic acid or rhodanine stain) or quantitative histochemistry (atomic absorption spectrophotometry) with normal serum ceruloplasmin levels; (9) dissecting (helter skelter) fibrosis of liver lobules; (10) macrovesicular and microvesicular fat in the absence of recent steroid therapy or significant hypoalbuminemia. Using a scoring system with one point for each criterion, the diagnosis of ICC requires 8 points.

Detection of ICC in its early stages is of importance in studying the natural history and treatment of the disease. *D*-Penicillamine has given encouraging results in the early stages of ICC but no improvement was noted in the established cases [21].

Indian immigrants have moved to the Western world in relatively large numbers since the 1960s but only three cases of ICC have been reported [61, 62] and only one was born and raised in England, the only instance of ICC in a child born in the Western world. The paucity of ICC among Indian immigrants' children born and raised in Western countries may be due to lack of environmental factors.

Lefkowitch et al. [63] reported cirrhosis resembling ICC in 4 American siblings with family history of cirrhosis. Lack of recognition of ICC-like cirrhosis as one of the rare forms of cirrhosis in non-Indian population may be due to lack of familiarity with this entity.

A study [21] to determine whether ICC can be prevented by avoiding exposure to excessive copper is in progress at this time in defined geographic areas of India where the villagers are being educated to avoid the use of brass utensils for storing or boiling milk and water.

Acknowledgements

The author is grateful to Dr. A.M. Pradhan for useful discussion of their on-going project on ICC, Dr. A.G. Bhagwat for providing references and electronmicrographs (fig. 8, 9) and Prof. B.S. Raichur and his associates for providing liver biopsy slides on cases of ICC. The author thanks Ms. Joyce Jackson for typing the manuscript.

References

1   Susruta: Susruta Samhita, Uttar Tantra, Saraswati Pustakalaya, Kanpur, India, 1952, chap. 27, verse 15. (Quoted by Sur and Bhatti, [2].)
2   Sur, A.M.; Bhatti, A.: Indian childhood cirrhosis. An inherited disorder of tryptophan metabolism. Br. med. J. *ii:* 529–531 (1978).
3   Bhagwat, A.G.; Walia, B.N.S.; Koshy, A.; Banerjee, K.: Will the real Indian childhood cirrhosis please stand up? Cleveland Clin. Q. *50:* 323–337 (1983).

4   Sen, B.C.: Enlargement of the liver in children. Transactions of the Calcutta Medical Society. Indian med. Gaz. *22:* 338–343 (1887).

5   Radhahrishna Rao, M.V.: Histopathology of liver in infantile biliary cirrhosis. Indian J. med. Res. *23:* 69–90 (1935).

6   Liver Disease Sub-Committee, Indian Council of Medical Research: Infantile cirrhosis of liver in India. Indian J. med. Res. *43:* 723–747 (1955).

7   Smetana, H.F.; Hadley, G.G.; Sirsat, S.M.: Infantile cirrhosis. An analytic review of the literature and a report of 50 cases. Pediatrics, Springfield *28:* 107–127 (1961).

8   Nayak, N.C.; Visalakshi, S.; Singh, M.; et al.: Indian childhood cirrhosis. A re-evaluation of its pathomorphologic features and their significance in the light of clinical data and natural history of the disease. Indian J. med. Res. *60:* 246–259 (1972).

9   Parekh, S.R.; Patel, B.D.: Epidemiologic survey of Indian childhood cirrhosis. Indian Pediat. *9:* 431–439 (1972).

10 Portmann, B.; Tanner, M.S.; Mowat, A.P.; et al.: Orcein-positive liver deposits in Indian childhood cirrhosis. Lancet *i:* 1338–1340 (1978).

11 Tanner, M.S.; Portmann, B.; Mowat, A.P.; et al.: Increased copper concentration in Indian childhood cirrhosis. Lancet *i:* 1203–1205 (1979).

12 Popper, H.; Goldfischer, S.; Sternlieb, I.; et al.: Cytoplasmic copper and its toxic effects-studies in Indian childhood cirrhosis. Lancet *i:* 1205–1208 (1979).

13 Bhagwat, A.G.; Vashisht, K.K.; Walia, B.N.S.: Clinicopathological and Ultrastructural studies in the siblings of Indian childhood cirrhosis. Fed. Proc. *39:* 877 (1980).

14 Bhave, S.A.; Pandit, A.N.; Pradhan, A.M.; et al.: Liver disease in India. Archs Dis. Childh. *57:* 922–928 (1982).

15 Achar, S.T.; Raju, B.V.; Sriramachari, S.: Indian childhood cirrhosis. J. Pediat. *57:* 744–758 (1960).

16 Bhagwat, A.G.: Indian childhood cirrhosis. Br. med. J. *284:* 194 (1982).

17 Anthony, P.P.; Ishak, K.G.; Nayak, N.C.; et al.: The morphology of cirrhosis. Definition, nomenclator and classification. Bull. Wld. Hlth Org. *55:* 521–540 (1977).

18 Bhagwat, A.G.: Indian childhood cirrhosis. Lancet *ii:* 640–641 (1979).

19 Tanner, M.S.; Portmann, B.: Indian childhood cirrhosis. Archs Dis. Childh. *56:* 4–6 (1981).

20 Nayak, N.C.; Sagreiya, K.; Ramalingaswami, V.: Indian childhood cirrhosis. The nature and significance of cytoplasmic hyaline of hepatocytes. Archs Path. *88:* 631–637 (1969).

21 Pandit, A.N.; Bhave, S.A.: Copper and Indian childhood cirrhosis. Indian Pediat. *20:* 893–898 (1983).

22 Pradhan, A.M.: Personal commun. (1984).

23 Nayak, N.C.; Ramalingaswami, V.: Indian childhood cirrhosis. Clin. Gastroenterol. *4:* 333–349 (1975).

24 Chandra, R.K.: Indian childhood cirrhosis. Genealogy data, alpha-foetoprotein, hepatitis antigen and circulating immune complexes. Trans. R. Soc. trop. Med. Hyg. *70:* 296–301 (1976).

25 Agarwal, S.S.; Lahori, V.C.; Mehta, S.K.; et al.: Inheritance of Indian childhood cirrhosis. Hum. Hered. *29:* 82–88 (1979).

26 Daniel, O.; Nath, I.; Nayak, N.C.; et al.: Reduction of circulating T-lymphocytes in Indian childhood cirrhosis. Indian J. med. Res. *68:* 798–804 (1978).

27 Aikat, B.K.; Bhattacharya, T.; Walia, B.N.S.: Morphological features of Indian child-

hood cirrhosis. The spectrum of changes and their significance. Indian J. med. Res. *62:* 953–963 (1974).

28   Joshi, V.V.: Unpubl. observations.

29   Bhagwat, A.G.; Walia, B.N.S.: Indian childhood cirrhosis. A commentary. Indian J. Pediat. *48:* 433–437 (1980).

30   Pandit, A.N.: Proceeding of Workshop on ICC. Indian Pediat. *20:* 741–746 (1983).

31   Nayak, N.C.; Ramalingaswami, V.; Roy, S.; et al.: Hepatitis-B virus and Indian childhood cirrhosis. Lancet *ii:* 109–111 (1975).

32   Salaspuro, M.; Sipponen, P.: Demonstration of an intracellular copper-binding protein by orcein staining in lon-standing cholestatic liver disease. Gut *17:* 787–790 (1976).

33   Roy, S.; Ramalingaswami, V.; Nayak, N.C.: An ultrastructural study of the liver in Indian childhood cirrhosis with particular reference to the structure of cytoplasmic hyaline. Gut *12:* 693–701 (1971).

34   Patel, B.D.; Parekh, S.R.; Chitale, A.R.: Pathology of Indian childhood cirrhosis with special emphasis on ultrastructural observations. XVth Int. Congr., International Academy of Pathology, Miami 1984.

35   Chuttani, H.K.; Sidhu, A.S.; Gupta, D.; et al.: Follow-up study of cases from Delhi epidemic of infectious hepatitis of 1955–56. Br. med. J. *ii:* 676–679 (1966).

36   Tanner, M.S.; Flower, A.J.E.; Bhave, S.A.; Pandit, A.N.: Does Indian childhood cirrhosis (ICC) result from viral infection in a copper-laden liver. Archs Dis. Childh. *23:* A922 (1982).

37   Suryanarayan Rao, K.; Madhavan, T.V.; Tulpule, P.G.: Incidence of toxigenic strains of Aspergillus flavus affecting ground nut crop in certain costal districts of India. Indian J. med. Res. *53:* 1196–1201 (1965).

38   Amala, I.; Kumari, S.; Screenivasamurthy, V.; et al.: Role of aflatoxin in Indian childhood cirrhosis. Indian Pediat. *7:* 262–270 (1970).

39   Yadgiri, B.; Reddy, V.; Tulpule, P.G.; et al.: Aflatoxin and Indian childhood cirrhosis. Am. J. clin. Nutr. *23:* 94–98 (1970).

40   Amla, I.; Kamala, C.S.; Gopalkrishna, G.S.; et al.: Cirrhosis in children from peanut meal contaminated by aflatoxin. Am. J. clin. Nutr. *24:* 609–614 (1971).

41   Chandra, R.K.: Immunological picture in Indian childhood cirrhosis. Lancet *i:* 537–540 (1970).

42   Chandra, R.K.; Chawla, V.; Verma, I.C.; et al.: Hepatitis-associated antigen and depressed cellular immunity in Indian childhood cirrhosis. Am. J. Dis. Child. *123:* 408–410 (1972).

43   Mehta, S.; Walia, B.N.; Ghai, O.P.; et al.: A qualitative study of plasma and urinary aminoacids in Indian childhood cirrhosis. Indian J. Pediat. *31:* 189–190 (1964).

44   Kapoor, S.K.; Singh, M.; Ghai, O.P.: Study of serum copper and copper oxidase in patients with Indian childhood cirrhosis. Indian J. med. Res. *59:* 115–121 (1971).

45   Goldfischer, S.; Popper, H.; Sternlieb, I.: The significance of variations in the distribution of copper in liver disease. Am. J. Path. *99:* 715–730 (1980).

46   Reed, G.B.; Butt, E.M.; Landing, B.H.: Copper in childhood liver disease. A histologic, histochemical and chemical survey. Archs Path. *93:* 249–255 (1972).

47   Tanner, M.S.; Kantarjian, A.H.; Bhave, S.A.; Pandit, A.N.: Early introduction of copper-contaminated animal milk feed as a possible cause of Indian childhood cirrhosis. Lancet *ii:* 992–995 (1983).

48   Weber, K.M.; Boston, R.C.; Leaver, D.D.: A kinetic model of copper metabolism in sheep. Aust. J. agric. Res. *31:* 773–790 (1980).

49   Banks, D.M.: Hereditary disorders of copper metabolism in Wilson's disease and Menke's disease; in Stanbury, Wyngaarden, Fredrickson, Goldstein, Brown, 'The metabolic basis of inherited disease'; 5th ed., pp. 1251–1268 (McGraw-Hill, New York 1983).

50   Camakaris, J.: Unpubl. results quoted in ref. 47.

51   Marwaha, N.; Nayak, N.C.; Roy, S.; et al.: The role of excess hepatic copper in the evolution of Indian childhood cirrhosis. Indian J. med. Res. *73:* 395–403 (1981).

52   Nayak, N.C.; Marwaha, N.; Kalra, V.; et al.: The liver in siblings of patients with Indian childhood cirrhosis. A light and electron microscopic study. Gut *22:* 295–300 (1981).

53   Dallner, G.; Siekevitz, P.; Palade, G.E.: Biogenesis of endoplasmic reticulum membranes. II. Synthesis of constitutive microsomal enzymes in developing rat hepatocytes. J. Cell Biol. *30:* 97–117 (1966).

54   Dallner, G.; Siekevitz, P.; Palade, G.E.: Biogenesis of endoplasmic reticulum membranes. I. Structural and chemical differentiation in developing rat hepatocytes. J. Cell Biol. *30:* 73–96 (1966).

55   Nayak, N.C.; Malaviya, A.N.; Chawla, V.; et al.: Alpha-fetoprotein in Indian childhood cirrhosis. Lancet *i:* 68–69 (1972).

56   Zeitzer, P.M.; Neerhout, R.C.; Fonkalsrun, E.W.; et al.: Differentiation between neonatal hepatitis and biliary atresia by measuring serum alphafetoproteins. Lancet *i:* 373–375 (1974).

57   Krishnamachari, K.A.V.R.; Bhat, R.V.; Nagarajan, V.; et al.: Hepatitis due to aflatoxicosis. An outbreak in Western India. Lancet *i:* 1061–1063 (1975).

58   Tandon, V.N.; Krishnamurthy, L.; Koshy, A.; et al.: Study of an epidemic of jaundice in Northwest India presumably due to toxic hepatitis. Gastroenterology *72:* 488–494 (1977).

59   Tandon, H.D.; Tandon, B.N.; Tandon, R.P.: A pathological study of the liver in an epidemic outbreak of veno-occlusive disease. Indian J. med. Res. *65:* 679–684 (1977).

60   Patel, B.D.; Parekh, S.R.; Chitale, A.R.: Histopathological evolution of Indian childhood cirrhosis. Indian Pediat. *14:* 19–28 (1974).

61   Tanner, M.S.; Portmann, B.; Mowat, A.P.; et al.: Indian childhood cirrhosis present in Britain with orcein-positive deposits in liver and kidney. Br. med. J. *iii:* 928–929 (1978).

62   Klass, H.J.; Kelly, J.K.; Warnes, T.W.: Indian childhood cirrhosis in the United Kingdom. Gut *21:* 344–350 (1980).

63   Lefkowitch, J.H.; Honig, C.L.; King, M.E.; et al.: Hepatic copper overload and features of Indian childhood cirrhosis in an American sibship. New Engl. J. Med. *307:* 271–277 (1982).

V.V. Joshi, MD, FRC Path, Department of Pathology,
CHNJ, United Hospitals Medical Center,
Newark, NJ 07107 (USA)

Perspect. pediatr. Pathol., vol. 11, pp. 193–213 (Karger, Basel 1987)

Degenerative Leiomyopathy with Massive Megacolon

Myopathic Form of Chronic Idiopathic Intestinal Pseudo-Obstruction Occurring in Indigenous Africans

Ronald O.C. Kaschula[a], *Sidney Cywes*[b], *Arnold Katz*[c], *Jan H. Louw*[d]

[a] Head, Pathology Laboratories, Red Cross War Memorial Children's Hospital, Cape Town; [b] Professor of Paediatric Surgery, Red Cross War Memorial Children's Hospital and University of Cape Town; [c] Consultant Paediatric Surgeon, Red Cross War Memorial Children's Hospital, Groote Schuur Hospital, and University of Cape Town; [d] Emeritus Professor of Surgery and former Head of Surgery at Groote Schuur Hospital, Red Cross War Memorial Children's Hospital, and University of Cape Town, South Africa

Introduction

Massive megacolon without aganglionosis, known as Bantu pseudo-Hirschsprung's disease, affects indigenous African children of southern, central, and east Africa [1], resembling a similar, but familial syndrome manifesting as non-propulsive colon [2]. Apart from gross colonic dilatation progressively extending proximally from the anal verge, no associated abnormality had been reported until 1976 [3]. The condition had been considered to be a functional anomaly of the autonomic nervous system which mainly afflicted the gastro-intestinal tract and occasionally the genito-urinary system. Identification of smooth muscle abnormalities makes degenerative leiomyopathy (DL) an appropriate term for this form of hollow viscus myopathy encountered in Africa.

Clinical Data

The Pathology Department records of Red Cross War Memorial Children's Hospital and Groote Schuur Hospital in Cape Town contain 25 cases of gross megacolon unassociated with mechanical obstruction (ano-rectal membrane) or aganglionosis during the 25-year period from 1955

Table I. Clinical presentation

Case no.	Year first seen	Sex	Age years	Gaseous distension of abdomen	Chronic constipation	Abdominal discomfort with cramps	Diarrhoea and vomiting	Dilatation of bladder/ureters	Megaduodenum	Dilated oesophagus
1	1955	M	8							
2	1956	F	10							
3	1960	M	14	+	+	+				
4	1960	M	3							
5	1960	M	19							
6	1962	F	7	+	+	+			+	
7	1963	F	10							
8	1964	M	7	+	+			+		
9	1969	M	7	+	+	0	+			
10	1971	F	11	+		0	+			
11	1972	M	10							
12	1973	M	4	+			+			
13	1974	M	11	+			+	+		+
14	1974	M	6	+		+				
15	1974	F	5	+						
16	1975	F	12							
17	1975	F	8	+	+	0	+			
18	1976	F	10	+	+	+	+			
19	1976	F	10	+		+	+		+	
20	1978	F	14							
21	1979	M	15	+				+	+	+
22	1979	M	7	+		0		+	+	+
23	1979	F	5	+	+	0	+			
24	1980	F	7	+		0	+			
25	1980	M	12	+	+	+				

+=Feature present; 0=feature absent.

through 1980. All were indigenous Africans (14 males and 11 females) with a mean age of 9½ (3–19) years when first undergoing a colonic or rectal biopsy (table I).

Each child was studied radiographically with chest and abdominal plain films and barium enemas and with colonic or rectal biopsies with full

Increased anal tone	Ano rectal mano-metry	Previous mal-nutri-tion	Previous tuber-culosis	Other remarks
				intestinal volvulus, perforation, septicaemia, and necropsy
			+	sigmoid colectomy followed by adhesions and obstruction
				anal sphincterotomy, scabies
				colonic resection followed by adhesions and obstruction
		+		parotid gland swelling
+	+	+	+	anal stretch, laparotomy followed by adhesions
+			+	hepatomegaly and intestinal malabsorption
				tap water enemas given by family
		+		colectomy followed by adhesions and obstruction, rickets, died
				laparotomy for volvulus, necrotizing entercolitis, died, necropsy
0	+		+	volvulus of caecum, episodes of haematuria
+			0	given repeated colonic washouts to remove impacted faeces
0		+		volvulus of colon, colectomy, died, necropsy, bladder fibrosis
0	+			lack of oesophageal peristalsis, laparotomy
0	+			recurrent symptoms refractory to all forms of treatment
0	+	+	+	tuberculosis in family
0	+			visible peristalsis

thickness of the muscularis propria including Auerbach's plexus. Submuco-sal suction biopsies were obtained from 12 cases (2 anal and 10 rectal) who had first been seen subsequent to 1972. After 1972, all specimens were studied by electron microscopy and histochemically. Manometric pressure studies of the anal sphincters were determined in 6 cases after 1976.

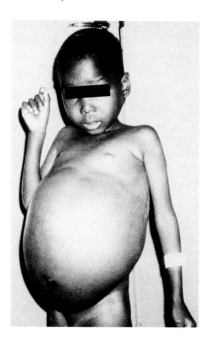

Fig. 1. Gross abdominal distension. Case 22, 7-year-old male.

From a retrospective study of the available bedside records of 17 cases, all (100%) had long-standing gaseous distension of the abdomen, often beginning in infancy (table I). The high order of abdominal distension simulated the late stage of pregnancy (fig. 1). Although 9 patients (53%) had episodes of diarrhoea, with or without vomiting, that frequency is not excessive in our patients. Eight of the 17 cases (47%) had chronic constipation for longer than 1 year, most often dating from early infancy. Six patients (35%) had episodes of abdominal discomfort, apparently with cramping pain, and another 6 patients (35%) had no pain at all.

Severe, non-uniform dilatation of rectum and colon with gas was often associated with impacted faeces. Of 6 patients with dilatation of oesophagus, duodenum, bladder, and ureters, the findings were confirmed at necropsy in 2. Although digital examination of the rectum in 3 cases revealed slight increase in anal tone, anorectal manometric studies in 6 cases revealed none with the spastic pattern of Hirschsprung's disease, but neither did they have the normal prompt relaxation response to stimulation by momentarily increasing intra-anorectal pressure.

Four children had been malnourished during earlier life, and 5 had previously been treated for tuberculosis. During the time that the children were under medical treatment, 3 of them had volvulus (1 child once of the small intestine, 1 child twice of the transverse colon, and 1 child twice of the caecum). Two children required repeated laparotomies to lyse adhesions causing recurrent intestinal obstruction following initial colonic resection. The overall experience with resection of grossly dilated colon and terminal ileum was most discouraging, since symptoms were not alleviated, and, if anything, surgery tended to hasten the progress of the disease.

Morphological Changes in Surgical Resections

Macroscopic

Of the partially resected colon or terminal ileum in 11 cases, the dilatation was usually much greater than in the megacolon due to Hirschsprung's disease but without muscle hypertrophy of the dilated segment, although muscle wall thickness varied. Following colonic resections several children required further surgical procedures to free adhesions causing intestinal obstruction. The post-resection dilatation of the colon and small intestines had progressed to involve a greater portion of the gut, although the most extensive muscle degeneration and fibrosis always affected the distal segments of the gastro-intestinal tract. After long-standing disease the serosal surface of the dilated colon and lower ileum sometimes had flattened fibrous plaques.

Microscopic

Specimens of colon and intestine had a consistent interstitial and intracellular oedema of the muscularis propria, less often of the muscularis mucosae, more prominent in the proximal sections of bowel, suggesting that it occurs relatively early in the evolution of the disease. Extracellular oedema was most conspicuous in the circular layer, while intracellular oedema, degeneration of muscle cells, and fibrous replacement of muscle was most obvious in the longitudinal layer of muscularis propria (fig. 2a, b). Degenerative changes in muscularis mucosae and both layers of muscularis propria tended to distribute focally or in alternating waves along the longitudinal axis of the muscle (fig. 3). The muscle cell cytoplasm was homogeneous and deeply eosinophilic; most nuclei were shrunken and

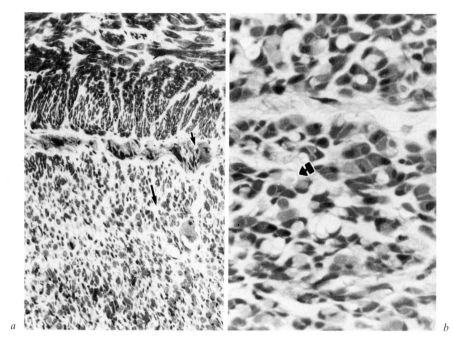

Fig. 2. Colonic muscularis. *a* Ganglia of Auerbach's plexus (short arrow) and separation of thinned and degenerate smooth muscle fibres of circular layer (long arrow). Case 10, 11-year-old female. Trichrome stain. ×100. *b* Degeneration with vacuolation (arrow) of muscle fibres. Case 19, 10-year-old female. HE. ×400.

pyknotic, although a few were slightly swollen and lightly eosinophilic, giving a superficial resemblance to a viral inclusion (fig. 4). With advancement of the degeneration, the muscle cells eventually disappeared, to be replaced by fibrosis. In the advanced lesion, alternating bands of fibrous tissue and muscle fibres were most striking in the outer longitudinal layer, less so in the circular layer and the muscularis mucosae. With progressive degeneration of the intervening segments of surviving muscle, a thick fibrous plaque extended to the serosa.

Of the 25 cases, 13 were free of inflammation, but 12 had an inflammatory cell infiltration confined to the muscularis propria in 6 cases, extending to mucosa and submucosa in 4 cases and to serosa and subserosa in 2 cases. Lymphocytes were the predominant inflammatory cell type accompanied by a few macrophages, eosinophils, and polymorphonuclear

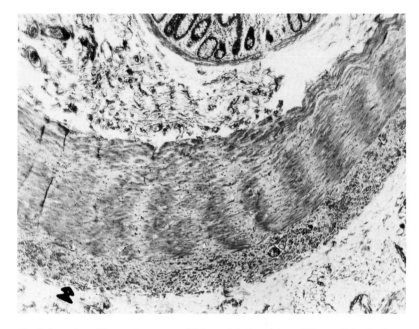

Fig. 3. Intestine. Alternating waves of light and dark staining of fibres of circular layer of muscularis propria. There is atrophy and separation of the muscle fibres of the longitudinal layer (arrow). Case 21, 15-year-old male. HE. ×25.

leucocytes. The focal inflammatory lesions in the muscularis were mainly localized to the circular layer of muscle, but infiltrating some ganglia of Auerbach's plexus in 3 cases without perceptible degenerative changes in the neurones or their supporting cells. Stains for tubercle bacilli and parasites were consistently negative. The neuronal cells in the ganglia of the intermyenteric and submucosal plexuses were normal.

Auerbach's intermuscular plexus and Meissner's submucosal plexus were displaced from their normal sites in 14 of the 25 cases. Several intermuscular ganglia lay within the middle third of the circular layer of muscle rather than in their usual position between the circular and longitudinal layers. Although minor displacement of ganglia of Auerbach's plexus to the outer third of the circular layer is a fairly frequent occurrence in colon and appendix of normal individuals, in this form of megacolon the displacement occurred three times as frequently and further away from the normal sites than in normal colons.

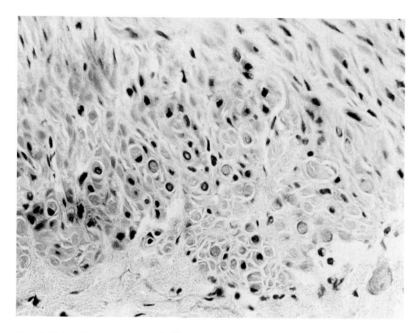

Fig. 4. Colon. Degenerate muscle fibres of muscularis propria with pyknotic nuclei as well as enlarged swollen nuclei containing homogeneous eosinophilic nucleoplasm. Case 13, 11-year-old male. HE. ×256.

The ganglia of Meissner's plexus were displaced into the centre of a slightly thickened muscularis mucosae in 1 of the 14 cases with displacement of Auerbach's ganglia to the central zone of the circular layer of muscle (fig. 5). Evaluation of the thin muscularis externa for displacement of ganglia is imprecise, since dilatation of bowel further narrows this already thin layer. Nevertheless, in 2 of the 14 cases with displaced Auerbach's ganglia, ganglion cells were also displaced into the central zone of the longitudinal layer.

Autopsy Findings

In autopsies performed on 3 of the 25 cases (cases 3, 17, and 21) the findings included gross dilatation of the intestines and structural changes in several small muscular arteries of the lung, spleen, liver, and kidney. Affected arteries had asymmetrical thickening of the intima with narrowing of the lumen due to proliferation of myofibroblasts and endothelial

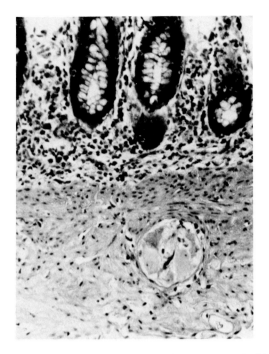

Fig. 5. Rectum. A ganglion of Meissner's plexus sited in the centre of thickened muscularis mucosa. Case 11, 10-year-old male. HE. ×125.

cells, accumulation of mucopolysaccharides, and deposition of collagen and reticulin fibres. The media was much attenuated due to changes in muscle cells, similar to that in the smooth muscle of gut wall. The surviving muscle of the media had alternating bands of densely eosinophilic and pale vacuolated cytoplasm in coronary arteries (fig. 6), submeningeal cerebral arteries, a pancreatic artery, and soft palate arteries. Medial fibrosis extended into an expanded adventitia.

Fibrous replacement of smooth muscle was a striking feature in the oesophagus, ureters, and urinary bladder of 1 case (No. 21). Interstitial and intracellular oedema occurred diffusely in both layers of muscularis propria of the oesophagus and focally in the ureters and urinary bladder. Alternating waves of muscle degeneration affected the oesophagus, but not ureters and bladder.

No abnormalities of the autonomic nervous system or of the central nervous system were identified. In case 3 the terminal event was peritonitis

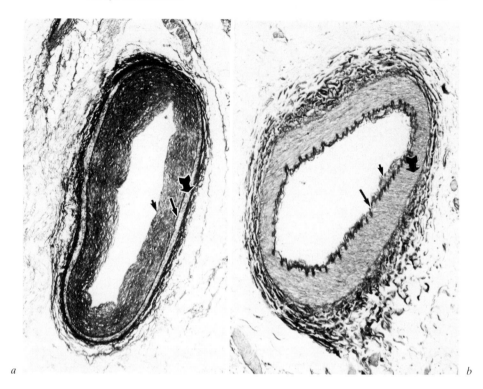

a   *b*

Fig. 6. Circumflex branch of left coronary artery. *a* Case 21, 15-year-old male, showing fibrous thickening of intimal layer (short arrow) with a thin, linear internal elastic lamina (long arrow) and a very thin, atrophic muscular layer (thick arrow). *b* An age-matched control coronary artery showing limited focal fibrous heaping of intimal layer (short arrow), a thick-folded internal elastic lamina (long arrow), and a normal muscular layer (thick arrow). Elastic van Gieson's stain. ×25.

following colonic resection; in case 17 it was necrotizing enterocolitis with septicaemia; and case 21 had a severe metabolic disturbance following an ileostomy and suffered a sudden cardiorespiratory arrest.

Histochemical Studies

Autonomic Nervous System
Anorectal mucosal biopsies for the evaluation of acetylcholinesterase activity of the autonomic nervous system of the gut were secured from 13

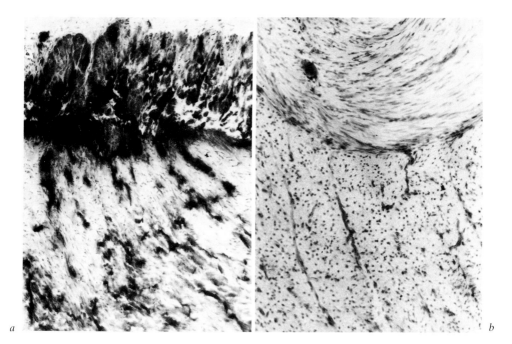

a
b

Fig. 7. Rectal muscularis propria. *a* Thick acetylcholinesterase-producing nerve fibrils have indistinct and smudgy borders. Case 24, 7-year-old female with massive megacolon. Stained by the technique of Lake et al. [5]. ×40. *b* Control case of aganglionic neuronal intestinal dysplasia as described by Schärli and Meier-Ruge [6], showing thin acetylcholinesterase-producing nerve fibrils with sharply defined borders. Lake's stain. ×63.

patients. Frozen sections were cut and stained according to the methods of Meier-Ruge et al. [4] and Lake et al. [5]. In 9 of these 13 cases additional tissue comprising the full thickness of the gut wall was used to study Auerbach's plexus using the same staining techniques.

None of the biopsies or resections studied had the overgrowth of long, thin acetylcholinesterase-containing nerve fibrils in the lamina propria and muscularis mucosae characteristic of the aganglionic segment of Hirschsprung's disease. Scanty, short, stubby acetylcholinesterase-containing fibrils occupied the lamina propria of 3 cases. In 2 of the 3 cases (Nos. 18 and 25) the fibrils were identified in continuity with ganglion cells, interpreted as axonal and dendritic extensions of abnormally placed nerves. Normal acetylcholinesterase-containing nerve cells and fibrils oc-

cupied the submucosa around submucosal vessels of all 3 cases. No case
had an increased number of ganglion cells in either the submucosal or intermyenteric plexuses.

Acetylcholinesterase activity of Auerbach's plexus and adjoining
muscularis propria evaluated in 9 cases showed normal enzyme activity in
the ganglia of Auerbach's plexus and an excessive number of thick, stubby
nerve fibrils amongst the muscle fibres of the circular and longitudinal
layers (fig. 7). This network of enzyme-containing nerve fibrils was not
quite as rich as that in the aganglionic segment of Hirschsprung's disease
or in neuronal intestinal dysplasia [6]. In both conditions there is imperfect
peristalsis in the terminal segments of rectum and colon having an abnormally rich network of acetylcholinesterase-containing nerve fibrils in mucosa, muscularis mucosae and muscularis propria. In Hirschsprung's disease the abnormal segment is aganglionic, whereas in neuronal intestinal
dysplasia the colon has normal ganglion cells. In DL, the border of the
thick, stubby nerve fibrils is indistinct as compared with the sharp border
in aganglionosis and in neuronal intestinal dysplasia. The intensity and
richness of this nerve plexus in DL is not uniform either with a single patient or among a group of patients, impairing its usefulness as a diagnostic
criterion.

Silver impregnation of thick frozen sections in 2 cases revealed the
same pattern of short, thick, and stubby nerve fibrils in the muscularis
propria as with the acetylcholinesterase stains. Although ganglia in Auerbach's plexus were argyrophilic, they were slightly fewer than normal.

Mucosal Enzyme Studies

In frozen sections of the mucosa of small and large intestines from 2
cases, acid and alkaline phosphatase and leucine aminopeptidase activities
were normal.

Muscle Enzyme Studies

In frozen sections of the muscularis propria of the colon of 4 cases,
adenosine triphosphatase activity and nicotine adenine dinucleotide tetra-
zolium reductase activity were normal.

Electron Microscopy

Colonic biopsy specimens from 7 patients were examined by electron
microscopy after fixation in buffered glutaraldehyde, embedding in
Spurr's resin, and staining with uranyl acetate and lead citrate.

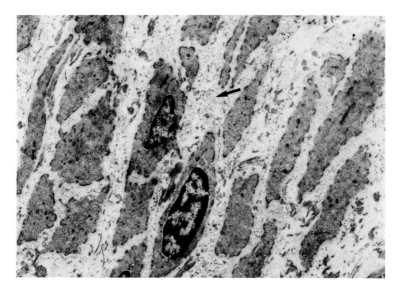

Fig. 8. Electron micrograph of a transverse section of colonic muscularis propria. Collagen fibres (arrow) and oedema fluid separate the atrophic muscle cells. They are small relative to the size of nuclei and collagen fibres. Case 11, 10-year-old male. ×6,800.

In the areas of muscle atrophy and oedema seen by light microscopy, the muscle fibres were reduced in size and widely separated by fluid and connective tissue containing collagen fibres (fig. 8). The atrophic fibres showed margination of nuclear chromatin, discontinuous or indistinct cytoplasmic membranes, and loss of pinocytotic vesicles. As a constant feature in less severely affected areas, fluid accumulated diffusely within the cytoplasmic membrane (fig. 9), sometimes manifest as multiple small vesicles just internal to the cytoplasmic membrane (fig. 10). The autopsy specimens of case 21 contained a scattering of thickened myofilaments as well as normal-sized myofilaments. No viral particles or crystalline deposits were encountered.

Discussion

Etiology, Pathogenesis, and Differential Diagnosis
The syndrome of DL clinically manifesting as massive megacolon and apparently occurring exclusively in young indigenous Africans was first

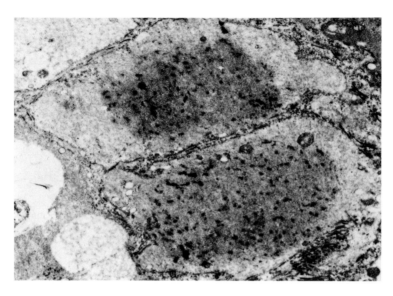

Fig. 9. Electron micrograph of a transverse section of colonic muscularis propria, show-ing paucity of pinocytotic vesicles, indistinct cytoplasmic membranes, and accumulation of fluid immediately internal to the cytoplasmic membrane. Case 24, 7-year-old female. ×10,500.

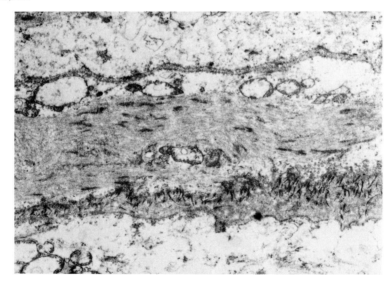

Fig. 10. Electron micrograph of longitudinal section of colonic muscularis propria showing vesicular accumulation of fluid immediately internal to the cytoplasmic membrane. Case 21, 15-year-old male. ×10,500.

recognized by Katz [1] who described 4 black children with the syndrome and called the syndrome Bantu pseudo-Hirschsprung's disease. The syndrome is characterized by a long history of increasing abdominal distension, features of obstruction, and massive megacolon extending down to the anorectal junction; no deficiency or abnormality of ganglion cells and no local obstruction or anal spasm or stenosis.

Although the aetiology of DL remains obscure, the morphological and functional defects are considered to be postnatal events. The youngest child was 3 years old, and, apart from 1 exception, symptoms in all cases began after the 2nd birthday. The disease has not affected family members in our cases, although a possible hereditary background is recorded by Hamilton et al. [7]. No association with congenital anomalies has been found. The predilection for indigenous Africans in east, central, and southern Africa suggests hereditary and cultural-environmental causes.

Similar syndromes of chronic idiopathic intestinal pseudo-obstruction (CIIP) have been described in the United States and Europe, where the majority of cases have been familial, suggesting a hereditary pattern [8–21]. CIIP is also characterized by repeated episodes of intestinal obstruction in the absence of an anatomic blockage of the intestinal lumen. Some patients with CIIP have a mild form of disease, suggesting a dominant trait of variable penetrance [8, 10–12].

CIIP has been associated with a large number of diseases including the abuse of laxatives [13–15, 22]. From among 27 patients with chronic intestinal pseudo-obstruction, Schuffler et al. [13] identified progressive systemic sclerosis, multiple jejunal diverticula, sclerosing mesenteritis, and various other forms of CIIP. None of our patients had Raynaud's phenomenon, the skin changes of systemic sclerosis, or intestinal diverticula. Although some patients had plaque-like areas of serosal fibrosis on their ileum and colon, none had inflammatory granulomas. None of our patients had the mucosal melanosis or hypertrophy of the muscularis mucosae identified in abusers of laxatives in western societies.

Based on CIIP as a clinical syndrome caused by ineffective intestinal propulsion, disorders of smooth muscle and the autonomic nervous system are most frequently implicated [19]. The myopathic form of the disorder is characterized by degeneration and fibrosis of smooth muscle and may be familial or sporadic in occurrence [9, 13, 17, 23]. Smooth muscle has a vacuolar degeneration with fragmentation and dropout, together with thinning and fibrosis of either the longitudinal muscle alone or both muscle layers. Damaged muscle cells have discontinuous plasma membranes with loss of alignment of the contractile filaments, vacuolated mitochondria, and electron lucency of cytoplasm [9]. The 7 cases of DL that we examined were similar to reported cases of hollow viscus myopathy, having disrupted cytoplasmic membranes and abnormal myofilaments. However, our cases did not have vacuolated mitochondria, and cytoplasmic electron lucency was localized to the circumferential area immediately beneath the plasma membrane of the smooth muscle cells. The accumulation of fluid within smooth muscle cytoplasm has been attributed to damaged plasma membranes allowing calcium and other cations to enter cell cytoplasm [7]. Our cases had no crystalline deposits. Affected colonic smooth muscle examined by atomic absorption spectrometric analysis from 1 of our patients revealed a slight excess of zinc, perhaps related to a zinc-containing ointment used on his skin.

Three neuropathic forms of CIIP have been reported [8, 20, 25]. A familial form affected 2 siblings with diffuse degenerative changes of the myenteric plexuses of oesophagus, small intestine, and colon. The neurons were reduced in number, and about one third contained round, eosinophilic, intranuclear, nonviral inclusions [8] also found in other neurones of the nervous system. The intestinal smooth muscle was normal. Another familial form affected 4 siblings who had mental retardation, calcifications of basal ganglia, and intestinal pseudo-obstruction attributed to degeneration of myenteric plexus [25]. A sporadic neuropathic form of CIIP has a destructive lesion of the myenteric plexuses of small intestine and colon [19, 20]. As the lesion cannot be demonstrated by conventional histological techniques, requiring silver impregnations of sections cut parallel to bowel wall, it is probably infrequently recognized. With the silver staining technique on 2 of our cases, we were unable to demonstrate significant loss of neurones or severe swelling or shrinkage of neurones. We interpret the shortening and thickening of axonal fibrils, with reduced number of axons and dendrites, as consequences of stretching of the myenteric plexus by the massive megacolon.

Another syndrome of functional intestinal obstruction described by Tanner et al. [21] becomes manifest shortly after birth. There is hypergangliosis with excessive immaturity of the neuronal cells (neuroblasts), no perceptible changes in the smooth muscle of the gut, and a characteristic lack of argyrophilic neurons. In addition there are short small intestine, malrotation, and pyloric hypertrophy. Symptoms in our cases were not evident until long after birth, nor was there hypergangliosis or neuronal immaturity in autonomic nervous system. Although the 2 cases in our series that were studied for argyrophilia did not have a normal pattern, neither did they have the absence or markedly reduced staining which characterizes functional intestinal obstruction.

Each of 3 autopsy cases of DL had vascular lesions affecting many small arteries bearing some resemblance to the vascular changes that occur in mixed connective tissue disease (MCTD) in childhood [26]. In MCTD there are overlapping clinical features of systemic lupus erythematosus, dermatomyositis, and scleroderma with high titres of antinuclear antibodies (speckled pattern) and antibodies directed against the ribonucleoprotein fraction of extractable nuclear antigen. Widespread proliferative vascular lesions include intimal proliferation, medial vessel wall thickening, plasma cell infiltration, fibrinoid degeneration, and fibrosis in the absence of hypertension. Some cases have membranous glomerulonephritis with vascular sclerosis. Intestinal pseudo-obstruction and megacolon are not features of MCTD, although hyaline material may replace gastro-intestinal muscle. Although the 3 autopsy cases of DL had diffuse vascular lesions with intimal proliferation and narrowing of lumina, there was some loss of media, no plasma cell infiltration, fibrinoid degeneration, or glomerular lesions. Three living cases of DL did not have raised titres of speckled antinuclear antibodies or antiribonucleoprotein antibodies.

Inflammatory foci in about half the cases of DL could reflect a response to a primary infective agent or the high incidence of intercurrent infection and enterocolitis facilitated by the marked constipation. Although various viral and parasitic infections are common in the population in which DL occurs, *Trypanasoma cruzi*, which causes Chagas' disease and megacolon in South and Central America, is unknown in Africa. Progressive generalized leiomyositis, reported by Wang et al. [27], probably represents an auto-immune disease manifesting as recurrent ileus, diarrhoea, respiratory infections, and eczema, accompanied by an extensive round cell infiltration throughout the muscular layers of the duodenum and jejunum, with loss of smooth muscle cells in the gastro-intestinal tract, blood vessels, and lungs. The vacuolar degeneration of smooth muscle, megacolon, and proliferative vascular lesions of DL have not been reported in progressive generalized leiomyositis.

The striking pattern of the degenerative changes in smooth muscle in alternating waves along the long axis of the intestine has not been reported in other forms of CIIP (fig. 3). The identical myofibrillary degeneration of the smooth muscle of the gastro-intestinal tract and bladder accompanying reduced cardiac output or shock has been related to the combined effect of hypoxia, shock, and increased release of catecholamines which permits excessive absorption of calcium ions, leading to hypercontractility of smooth muscle and the formation of eosinophilic contraction bands [28]. Extending this hypothesis to DL, intimal proliferation with luminal narrowing of mesenteric arteries would enhance hypoxia of intestinal smooth muscle. Decreased mesenteric arterial blood flow in DL could thus account for the high incidence of wavy contraction bands which are not conspicuous in other types of CIIP. Excessive absorption of calcium ions into smooth muscle cells may also account for the marked vacuolation of the cells identified by both light and electron microscopy as well as the cytoplasmic crystalline deposits reported by Hamilton et al. [7].

The displacement of autonomic ganglia to sites deep in the muscle layers suggests a developmental anomaly. If the autonomic nervous plexus were a relatively rigid network and less compliant than the muscularis to excessive distension, the displacement could be secondary to the dilatation of the gut. In such an event the stubby outlines of the argyrophilic and acetylcholinesterase-producing nerves in the muscularis propria could also be a reaction to neuromuscular disruptions. The characteristic wavy segmental fibrosis interspersed with stretched degenerating muscle could represent the result of excessive mechanical stretching with loss of peristalsis. Since generalized degeneration of smooth muscle affects the genito-urinary tract and various muscular arteries, a primary mechanical mechanism of overdistension is an unlikely primary cause.

Environmental, nutritional, and cultural habits play major roles in disease patterns that have a high frequency in indigenous Africans in central and southern Africa. In almost all cultures native to this area, it is considered obligatory for children to defaecate at least once each day. Failure to do so often leads to administration of a herbal enema. Herbal enemas are also given for many other cultural reasons, such as to placate the ancestral spirits. Very few rural Africans will go through childhood without having several herbal enemas for one reason or another. The ingredients of the fluid administered in the enemas are extremely variable and cause mucosal ulceration when potassium permanganate is added in excessive amounts. Some of the herbal ingredients are lethal, causing liver and kidney failure [29, 30]. Toxic agents with the potential to cause vascular endothelial proliferation include pyrrolizidine alkaloids (responsible for causing Senecio poisoning) and Clostridium organisms. Various aloe extracts are the most frequent enema fluid ingredients administered to patients who develop DL. A toxin specifically affecting autonomic nerves and smooth muscle has not been demonstrated in these extracts, but a hypothetical toxin would account for the involvement of smooth muscle outside the gastro-intestinal tract, particularly in the muscular arteries. Aloes contain anthraquinones which are bowel irritants and when given parenterally are extremely potent cell poisons, even in minute doses [31]. Abuse of anthraquinone laxatives taken orally causes colonic melanosis, mucosal inflammation, hypertrophy of muscularis mucosae, atrophy of muscularis propria, and damage and loss of myenteric neurons [22]. As none of the cases of DL had melanosis and hypertrophy of muscularis mucosae, and as damage and loss of myenteric neurons were inconspicuous, extract of aloes in herbal enemas is unlikely as the sole cause.

Acknowledgements

This study has been supported by the Medical Research Council of South Africa, the Cape Provincial Administration, and the University of Cape Town, South Africa.

References

1   Katz, A.: Pseudo-Hirschsprung's disease in Bantu children. Archs Dis. Childh. *41:* 152–154 (1966).
2   Pages, R.; Duhamel, B.: Intrinsic non-propulsive colon. Archs Dis. Childh. *41:* 151–152 (1966).
3   Kaschula, R.O.C.: Some unusual neuromuscular disorders of the rectum and colon. Archs Dis. Childh. *52:* 514–515 (1977).
4   Meier-Ruge, W.; Lutterbeck, P.M.; Herzog, B.; Morger, R.; Moser, R.; Schärli, A.: Acetylcholinesterase activity in suction biopsies of the rectum in the diagnosis of Hirschsprung's disease. J. pediat. Surg. *7:* 11–17 (1972).
5   Lake, B.D.; Puri, P.; Nixon, H.H.; Claireaux, A.E.: Hirschsprung's disease: an appraisal of histochemically demonstrated acetylcholinesterase activity in suction rectal biopsy specimens as an aid to diagnosis. Archs Pathol. Lab. Med. *102:* 244–247 (1978).
6   Schärli, A.F.; Meier-Ruge, W.: Localized and disseminated forms of neuronal intestinal dysplasia mimicking Hirschsprung's disease. J. pediat. Surg. *16:* 164–170 (1981).
7   Hamilton, D.G.; Wainwright, H.C.; Isaacson, C.: Pathology of hereditary hollow visceral myopathy. Proc. XIIIth Int. Congr. Int. Acad. of Pathology, p. 47 (IAP, Paris 1980).
8   Schuffler, M.D.; Bird, T.D.; Sumi, S.M.; Cook, A.: A familial neuronal disease presenting as intestinal pseudo-obstruction. Gastroenterology *75:* 889–898 (1978).

9   Schuffler, M.D.; Lowe, M.C.; Bill, A.H.: Studies of idiopathic intestinal pseudo-obstruction. I. Hereditary hollow visceral myopathy: clinical and pathological studies. Gastroenterology 73: 327–338 (1977).

10   Schuffler, M.D.; Pope, C.E.: Studies of idiopathic intestinal pseudo-obstruction. II. Hereditary hollow visceral myopathy: family studies. Gastroenterology 73: 339–344 (1977).

11   Byrne, W.J.; Cipel, L.; Euler, A.R.; Halpin, T.C.; Ament, M.E.: Chronic idiopathic intestinal pseudo-obstruction syndrome in children. Clinical characteristics and prognosis. J. Pediat. 90: 585—594 (1977).

12   Teixidor, H.S.; Heneglian, M.A.: Idiopathic intestinal pseudo-obstruction in a family. Gastrointest. Radiol. 3: 91–95 (1978).

13   Schuffler, M.D.; Rohrmann, C.A.; Chaffee, R.G.; Brand, D.L.; Delany, J.H.; Young, J.H.: Chronic intestinal pseudo-obstruction. A report of 27 cases and review of the literature. Medicine 60: 173–196 (1981).

14   Hirsh, E.H.; Brandenburg, D.; Hersh, T.; Scott-Brooks, W.: Chronic intestinal pseudo-obstruction. J. clin. Gastroent. 3: 247–254 (1981).

15   Anuras, S.; Shirazi, S.S.: Colonic pseudo-obstruction. Am. J. Gastroent. 79: 525–532 (1984).

16   Faulk, D.L.; Anuras, S.; Christensen, J.: Chronic intestinal pseudo-obstruction. Gastroenterology 74: 922–931 (1978).

17   Faulk, D.L.; Anuras, S.; Gardner, G.D.; Mitros, F.A.; Summers, R.W.; Christensen, J.: A familial visceral myopathy. Ann. intern. Med. 89: 600–606 (1978).

18   Jacobs, E.; Ardichvili, D.; Perissino, A.; Gottiguies, P.; Hanssens, J.F.: A case of familial visceral myopathy with atrophy and fibrosis of the longitudinal muscle layer of the entire small bowel. Gastroenterology 77: 745–750 (1979).

19   Schuffler, M.D.; Jonak, Z.: Chronic idiopathic intestinal pseudo-obstruction caused by degenerative disorder of the myenteric plexus. Gastroenterology 82: 476–486 (1982).

20   Dyer, N.H.; Dawson, A.M.; Smith, B.F.; Todd, I.P.: Obstruction of bowel due to lesion in the myenteric plexus. Br. med. J. i: 686–689 (1969).

21   Tanner, M.S.; Smith, B.; Lloyd, J.K.: Functional intestinal obstruction due to deficiency of argyrophil neurones in the myenteric plexus. Familial syndrome presenting with short small bowel, malrotation and pyloric hypertrophy. Archs Dis. Childh. 51: 837–841 (1976).

22   Cummings, J.H.: Progress report. Laxative abuse. Gut 15: 758–766 (1974).

23   Schuffler, M.D.; Deitch, E.A.: Chronic idiopathic intestinal pseudo-obstruction. A surgical approach. Ann. Surg. 192: 752–761 (1980).

24   Smith, J.A.; Hauser, S.C.; Madara, J.L.: Hollow visceral myopathy. A light and electron microscopic study. Am. J. surg. Pathol. 6: 269–275 (1982).

25   Cocker, R.; Hill, E.E.; Rushton, D.I.; Smith, B.; Hawkins, C.F.: Familial steatorrhoea with calcification of the basal ganglia and mental retardation. Q. Jl Med. 42: 771–783 (1973).

26   Singsen, B.H.; Swanson, V.L.; Bernstein, B.H.; Heuser, E.T.; Hanson, V.; Landing, B.H.: A histologic evaluation of mixed connective tissue disease in childhood. Am. J. Med. 68: 710–717 (1980).

27   Wang, C.I.; Swanson, V.L.; Landing, B.H.: Progressive generalized leiomyositis: an autoimmune disease? Clin. res. 26: 174 (1978).

28 Renteria, V.G.; Fernandez, R.; Contreras, M.: Degeneración miofibrilar del musculo liso del tracto gastrointestinal y de la vejiga urinaria en pacientes con bajo gasto cardiaco. Archos Inst. Cardiol. Mexico *48:* 138–148 (1978).

29 Wainwright, J.; Schonland, M.M.: Toxic hepatitis in black patients in Natal. S. Afr. med. J. *51:* 571 (1977).

30 Wainwright, J.; Schonland, M.M.; Canday, H.A.: Toxicity of *Callilepis laureola*. S. Afr. med. J. *52:* 313 (1977).

31 Smith, B.: Pathology of cathartic colon. Proc. R. Soc. Med. *65:* 288 (1972).

Ronald O.C. Kaschula, MD, Head, Pathology Laboratories,
Red Cross War Memorial Children's Hospital, Cape Town (South Africa)

Subject Index

Abdominal pain, esophagitis 100
Acid reflux test 128, 129
Aflatoxin, Indian childhood cirrhosis 185
Alveolar lesions, bronchopulmonary
 dysplasia 22, 23
Aminoaciduria, Indian childhood cirrhosis
 185
Anemia
 gastroesophageal reflux 126
 iron-deficiency, idiopathic pulmonary
  hemosiderosis 48
Animal models, respiratory distress
 syndrome 7, 25–33
Antibodies, glomerular basement
 membrane 67
Apnea, gastroesophageal reflux 126
Arteriovenous fistula, spider-angioma
 type 89
Asthma, gastroesophageal reflux 126
Atelectasis, respiratory distress syndrome
 15
Autonomic nervous system, massive
 megacolon 203, 204

Bantu pseudo-Hirschsprung's disease,
 see Massive megacolon
Barium esophagram 100, 127
Barrett's esophagus 108–112, 142, 143
 columnar-lined mucosa, types 108
 diagnosis, biopsy site 110
 differential diagnosis 112
 mental retardation 111
Bethanecol, gastroesophageal reflux 143

Bilirubin, leakage, respiratory distress
 syndrome 18
Bone marrow transplant, gastroesophageal
 reflux 119
Bronchitis, gastroesophageal reflux 126
Bronchopulmonary dysplasia 7
 alveolar lesions 22, 23
 artificial ventilation 21
 bronchiolar lesions 22, 23
 diagnosis 25
 etiology 24
 pulmonary oxygen toxicity 23
 vs Wilson-Mikity syndrome 24, 25

Cardiac abnormalities, gastroesophageal
 reflux 127
Central nervous system disorders,
 gastroesophageal reflux 126
Chemotherapy
 esophagitis 120
 gastroesophageal reflux 120
Chronic idiopathic intestinal pseudo-
 obstruction 207, 208
 laxatives 207
 progressive systemic sclerosis 207
Cirrhosis
 Indian childhood, *see* Indian childhood
  cirrhosis
 liver, pulmonary arteriovenous fistulae
  89
Continuous positive airway pressure 6
Cow's milk allergy 64, 65
Cystic fibrosis, gastroesophageal reflux 120